A Vision for Plymouth

David Mackay
MBM Arquitectes

Roger Zogolovitch
Martin Harradine
AZ Urban Studio

Authors: David Mackay (MBM Arquitectes)
Roger Zogolovitch and Martin Harradine (AZ Urban Studio)

Editor: Kit Wedd

Design concept: Estudi Canó, Barcelona and Alex Casas

Designer: James Crisp, Document Production Centre,
University of Plymouth

Printed by: Deltor Communications Ltd.

Copyright: MBM Arquitectes/AZ Urban Studio/Plymouth 2020 © 2004

ISBN: 1-84102-124-5

Cover image: Abstracted structure of the Vision Plan

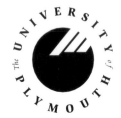

A Vision for Plymouth

Contents

7   **About the Authors**

7   **Acknowledgements**

9   **Foreword**

10 **Introduction**

13 **Chapter One: Principles of the Vision**
14   Recovering a lost tradition
16   The form of the public realm
21   The scale of enclosure
22   Movement through the public realm
24   The memory of place

29 **Chapter Two: The Development Approach**
30   The conditions
38   The opportunity

43 **Chapter Three: The MBM Vision for Plymouth**
44   Recovery of the waterfront city
48   Invigorating the Abercrombie Plan

51 **Chapter Four: The Elements of the Plan**
52   Millbay
61   The City Centre
71   Armada Way
75   Sutton Harbour
82   The Waterfront

89 **Chapter Five: Recommendations**
90   City-wide vision – connecting the opportunities
90   Population and economic growth
91   City management – responsibilities, strengths and weaknesses
92   Agencies, institutions and leadership
96   The wider context of the 'vision' strategy

100 **Image Credits**

A city must be so designed as to make its people at once secure and happy

Aristotle

About the Authors

David Mackay

David Mackay has been a partner at MBM Arquitectes for more than 45 years. Apart from many housing and school projects the team is probably best known for their masterplanning of the Olympic Village and Port in Barcelona in 1992. David was a member of the Senate Advisory Committee for the unification of Berlin, has served on many major competition juries, and is currently advisor to the Dublin Corporation. He has held a number of academic posts, most recently as Senior Design Fellow (2000 – 01) at the London School of Economics, Cities Programme. He has written several books and articles and lectures internationally on architecture and urban design. The Plymouth project was carried out with his partners Oriol Bohigas, Josep Martorell, Oriol Capdevila and Francesc Gual.

Roger Zogolovitch

Roger Zogolovitch is an architect and developer, and director of AZ Urban Studio. He has extensive experience of design-led development, and has led many large-scale urban projects in his career. His recent development, 1 Centaur Street, London, has won a number of leading architectural awards and received widespread critical acclaim as a major contribution to the current debate on urban housing. Roger has been closely involved in the leadership of both the Royal Institute of British Architects and the Architectural Association, and is currently a course director at the London School of Economics.

Martin Harradine

Martin Harradine is a principal consultant at AZ Urban Studio, where he has been since gaining a postgraduate degree from the London School of Economics, Cities Programme. He has managed a number of masterplanning and urban design projects, many in collaboration with MBM. Martin has previously worked in a number of built environment positions, ranging from a leading research project on the resurgence of urban tuberculosis to community planning education.

Acknowledgements

The Vision for Plymouth project was led and administered by the Plymouth 2020 Partnership and Plymouth City Council, both of whom provided exemplary support, input and resources throughout the duration of the project. Substantial funding for the study was provided by a range of local businesses and institutions, and without such civic support and belief the venture would not have been possible.

Special thanks and acknowledgement must be given to the support received from the University of Plymouth, which has both provided input into the project and embraced and accommodated its recommendations and principles in the development of their estate, which has a critical position within the city. The continued support and funding that the University of Plymouth has provided has made this publication possible, and the authors extend their greatest thanks.

Foreword

Plymouth's history is the history of opportunity. With its magnificent natural assets, enviable heritage and its skilled and creative population, Plymouth deserves an international reputation as one of Europe's finest maritime cities.

Out of the adversity of war we commissioned one of the foremost town planners, Patrick Abercrombie, to create a bold new vision for our city. Over the ensuing decades Plymouth may not have always realised that vision and, consequently, its full potential. We now stand on the brink of our greatest challenge since the war; namely to make Plymouth synonymous with the urban renaissance of England. Our aim is to make Plymouth a city of over 300,000 people so that it can take its place amongst the top ten cities in this country with all that will bring in terms of new shops, new community and cultural facilities and new homes.

David Mackay's bold and exciting new vision will help us achieve this. It has attracted widespread support and created a sense of real excitement. It builds upon some of the innovative planning and regeneration we had been undertaking in the last few years and brings a fresh international perspective with new ideas about how our city needs to evolve. The vision represents a step change of pace, intensity and quality of development in the city. It captures so well the opportunities for reviving our city centre and its links to the waterfront and surrounding areas. But with opportunity comes great challenge. Like all truly great visions it is aspirational, challenging, but deliverable. It asks Plymouth the fundamental question: what sort of city do you want to be? To achieve our vision we must think outside the box, create new partnerships, be bold, confident and ambitious, and also ensure that we involve the people of the city itself at every stage.

The vision has played an important role in developing the sense of optimism felt throughout the city at the moment. There is a sense that what we are doing now will affect future generations. It will play a crucial role not only in how the city sees itself, but also how the rest of the world sees it. Quite simply, history is being made. This is a huge responsibility but it is also a huge opportunity and one that we cannot afford to miss.

There is a buzz about Plymouth at the moment – and it is not just the hum of machinery on building sites. People stop each other in the street to talk about the changes they see around them. They are no longer on the sidelines and their interest in their own city has been revived. The vision requires much work to be done and its delivery, I am pleased to say, has already started with our project to transform Armada Way.

This book gives a sense of what Plymouth is all about and all that it will be. Once again we can be a city of opportunity and I hope you are as excited about the contribution this vision will play in making it happen. It is now time to deliver.

Councillor Tudor Evans
Leader of Plymouth City Council

Introduction

This publication outlines a vision for the future of Plymouth that has been developed by MBM Arquitectes, Barcelona,[1] and AZ Urban Studio, London.[2] The work presented here has emerged in response to a widely-held view across the community of institutions and businesses in Plymouth that a sea change in thinking about the city should be explored, and an overall spatial development strategy should be created that enables the potential of the city and its urban area to be fully realised.

The city image often suffers from a perception of urban decay and stagnation associated with the rigid rebuilding of the post-war City Centre, the overbearing nature of much of the road network, and the feeling that Plymouth simply isn't punching its weight. This combination of problems has led to sustained concern among key local stakeholders about the poor quality of the urban environment in and around the City Centre, and the lack of a clearly expressed strategic vision for the future to bring about change.

Through the leadership of Plymouth 2020 Partnership and Plymouth City Council, a brief to explore new thinking about the city and its future was generated. Plymouth 2020 Partnership commissioned MBM Arquitectes and AZ Urban Studio to produce a vision for the built environment of the central area of Plymouth that would address a set of specific objectives, namely:

- add value to existing thinking on strategic opportunity areas
- strengthen connections to the waterfront
- promote the interconnection of different communities and neighbourhoods
- provide opportunities for long-term growth
- improve the image of the city.

The preparation of this vision took several months, during which the authors were closely involved with the city and many of its citizens. The participation of officers of Plymouth City Council has been of great benefit to the work, as it has helped us to achieve a considered balance between visionary aspirations and deliverability. The input from local people has ensured that the ideas and approaches we recommend for Plymouth are not simply products imported from other cities across Europe and the rest of the world where they have been seen to work. Rather, they have emerged from a process of learning from both historical and contemporary experience, and have been selected and adapted to work within the particular context of Plymouth.

The vision is not a fixed blueprint for the exact future of the city but a review of strengths and weaknesses, an assessment of direction, a pointer to opportunity, and an invitation to aspire. The city, an artificial creation of civilisation, is a work of art that reshapes itself in response to various influences over time. Any work of human creation needs an author: Wren, Wood, Nash and Abercrombie are but a few of the authors of urban form who have left their mark on the English city. All cities, however, outlive their original authors and must adapt themselves to changing circumstances over time. Our proposals for the repair and transformation of Plymouth are soundly based on a close analysis of the form of the fragments of the city under study. Our method, in which the physical response of repair and transformation is grounded in an analysis of place, problems and opportunity, is designed to create proposals that are practical and deliverable.

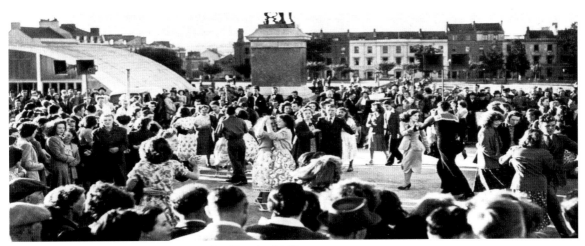

1. **People of Plymouth dancing on the Hoe in 1941**
Have we the chance to dance again?

Our process of developing a vision has involved capturing the essence of the city and using it to inform and shape the future.

- It is about discovering what works for Plymouth, and what is holding it back
- It is an opportunity to challenge perceptions and raise ambitions
- It invites citizens to engage and aspire
- It encourages new routes to delivery and achievement
- It provides a direction and driver for future change
- It informs the ongoing development and revision of statutory plans.

The vision presented here examines both the wider context of the city and the local conditions, and proposes a development and public space strategy for repairing the very heart of the City Centre, as a driver for the regeneration of Plymouth. It aims to deliver a string of coherent and legible public spaces, contained by buildings in scale with these spaces, which together will give form to the fragments of the city. This approach, when employed in other cities, has been shown to stimulate high-quality business, education, residential and recreation opportunities for citizens, investors, and visitors alike. These are the goals to which the Plymouth 2020 Partnership aspires.

This story of the vision is broadly structured in five chapters. The first explores the principles that underpin the approach taken to the city, providing examples of how they have been successfully employed in other cities. Chapter Two focuses on an analysis of the particularity of Plymouth, and presents a summarised context of the development opportunities that our vision emerges from and the constraints that it responds to. The third chapter describes the essence of our strategic vision for Plymouth; the individual elements of the plan are explored and explained in greater detail in Chapter Four. The concluding chapter recalls the recommendations for each area, presents possible routes to realising the vision and places this process and product of vision in the context of broader challenges facing the planning and development of cities throughout the United Kingdom.

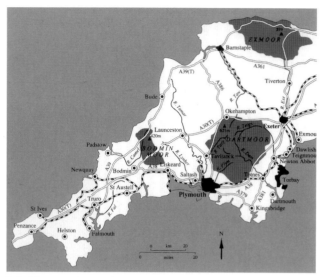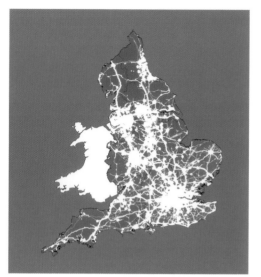

2, 3. **Plymouth: regional and national setting**
The city has an important relationship to a tranquil countryside

The vision has already been launched for discussion and consideration by all parties, and offered for consultation to the people of Plymouth. It will be tested and analysed by the relevant authorities, and subsequently inform the ongoing review and shaping of Council policy and strategy. Its impact on statutory plan making is vitally important, and there are already signs that some of the thinking embodied in the vision is being incorporated into Plymouth City Council policy. The scale of the opportunity and challenge outlined in the vision will probably require some form of 'delivery vehicle' to be set up to undertake key elements that the private sector alone will not deliver.

This book celebrates a process initiated by the RIBA conference 'Urban Plymouth... regeneration with inspiration' in 2002, which is now influencing development on the ground – a huge achievement within the UK planning system. This body of work is therefore relevant as an exemplary model of a process, led in the first instance by the private sector, and now adopted by the public sector. It should also be of interest and value to students and practitioners of urban design, architecture and planning, and of course, the people who live in, and love, Plymouth.

We believe that with support at all levels of public and private leadership, the vision outlined within this book can be realised at Plymouth over the next 20 years.

Notes

1. Josep Martorell, Oriol Bohigas, David Mackay, Oriol Capdevilla and Francesc Gual (Partners).

2. Roger Zogolovitch and Martin Harradine (Principals).

Chapter One
Principles of the Vision

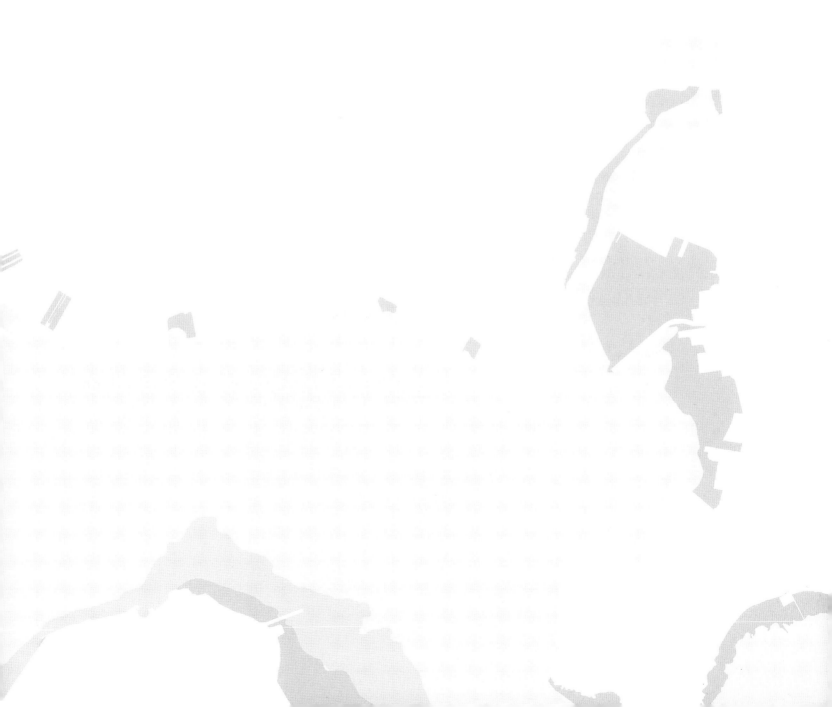

Recovering a lost tradition

In his ninepenny book, *Town Planning*, published in 1940,[1] Thomas Sharp begins by quoting D.H. Lawrence's description of English towns as 'a great scrabble of ugly pettiness over the face of land'. He allows Lawrence to continue, 'The English are town birds through and through. Yet they don't know how to build a city, how to think of one, or how to live in one. They are all suburban, pseudo-cottagers, and not one of them knows how to be truly urban. The English may be mentally and spiritually developed; but as citizens of splendid cities they are more ignominious than rabbits.'

Sharp quotes Lawrence in order to disagree with him. The English, he claims, 'once built towns which, according to the standards of their times, were excellent instruments for the living of a good social life; which were altogether *admirable essays in large-scale architectural composition*.' We have emphasised the last phrase because it describes the result of a process very different to the loss of confidence in town planning and consequent reliance on fragmentary proposals that Sharp observed among his contemporaries. Although made 65 years ago, his observations are worth repeating at length, as they remain the basis of the principles that have guided this vision for Plymouth in 2003.

> Right up till a hundred years ago there was a remarkably strong and virile town tradition in England. That tradition was very different from the continental tradition. It was none the worse for that. But it is a curious thing that today not only the ordinary citizen, not only writers like Lawrence, but our professional men whose job it is to study and build towns, our architects and town-planners, are mostly unaware that such a tradition ever existed, and are content to belaud foreign towns and sigh plaintively because we have never built in precisely the same way in England.

> Towns have sometimes been described as the physical expression of a nation's civilisation. The physical form of a town does in many ways reflect fairly accurately the social condition of the people who live in it, their mode of life, their cultural achievement, their economic status, the kind of government they possess. The town reflects those characteristics because it arises out of them. And it is, of course, precisely because of this that the English town tradition developed on its own individual lines.

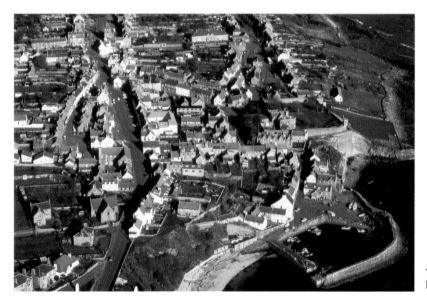

4. **Crail, Fife**
Planned through tradition

Our fall from grace has been very deep during the last century. We are not very sensible, however, because of that, to forget that we once did, in fact, live and build in grace. It is, indeed, all the more necessary for us to remember. The English contribution to the art of building towns was once an original and a valuable one. It is important that this should be realised, for if we are ever again to build good towns we shall need to restore our lost confidence, and perhaps to re-establish something of the old traditions.

The English town was, and is, characterised by being less dense than its continental counterpart. There was little traditional restraint to prevent expansion into the countryside – whether to provide manufacturing sites during the Industrial Revolution, suburban housing alongside the spreading Victorian railway network, or homes for heroes after the First World War. The traditional skills of English town-making were lost, so that the sudden need to rebuild cities after the Second World War gave rise to countless examples of bad planning.

Not that the generation charged with post-war reconstruction felt the need to rediscover old skills. Sixty years ago, when James Paton Watson, the city engineer, and Patrick Abercrombie, the eminent town planner, came together to produce their *Plan for Plymouth*,[2] they worked in heroic times. German air raids had destroyed both Devonport and the heart of the city itself. It was a brave gesture during the early days of the war to pave the way for the future. It was also during the heroic early days of town planning, a time when radical solutions were sought for the ills of the nineteenth century. On the ground cleared by the enemy's bombs the ideal of a healthy, functional city could become reality. Each area would have its specific function: there would be a place to dwell and sleep, a place for exercise and sport, a place for work, a place for culture, a place for the public administration and a place for commerce and shopping.

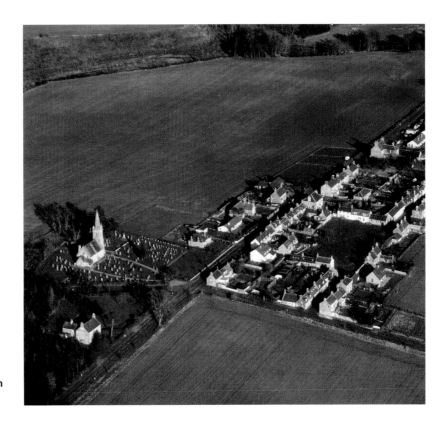

5. **Gavinton, East Lothian**
A planned village

Having separated these functions, or uses, the planner faced the task of providing transport between them. The obvious solution was the motor car. However, the police, alarmed by increasing numbers of road accidents, wished to separate pedestrians from traffic. Traffic engineers calculated for fast traffic in towns with wider roads, generous curves, hundreds of oddly-shaped 'traffic islands' – and eventually dealt with any unrepentant pedestrians by installing fences and railings along the edges of the road. The traditional role of the street as a meeting place was forgotten.

Today attitudes to urban life have changed. There is more respect for the past, and a greater desire to mix uses to generate local diversity. In spite of the demand for housing, more effort is made to discourage the expansion of the city into the countryside and to protect existing villages and towns from expansion. These changes have implications: if expansion is to be prevented, then empty pockets of land within the city must be identified and developed, and a reasonable increase in density must be encouraged. If social exclusion is to be avoided, then planners must provide better connections and places where people can meet. We need to find the right instruments to repair our urban environments, and the search begins with a re-examination of the quality of our public space.

The past of Plymouth gives us the key to the future, but it is a past that must be interpreted in the light of our own times. The juxtaposition of different architectural styles from different epochs is one of the delights of the historic high street. We must rediscover that delight by giving our own culture, today's culture, a chance to contribute to the streetscape. That culture is based on modernity – in other words, the ability to question everything constructively and not accept things just because they are there; it is a question of attitude, not style.

The form of the public realm

The street is of great consequence; it is important to us and must be treated with respect. The way in which we look after our streets clearly demonstrates our level of commitment to civilised society.

Anthropological research has revealed the deep-rooted importance of the street to different societies. In the earliest settlements of Mesopotamia, the first streets connected individual patio dwellings that were bounded by closely packed mud walls, and provided a link to the cultivated land beyond the settlement. Thus the street acquired a built form. Later, in Greek and Roman cities with more stratified societies and prosperous merchant and administrative classes, the appearance of building façades became socially important as an expression of influence and wealth, and this had consequences for the form of the street. The early street system established in Alexandria from 332 BC by the architect Dinocretes was based on an orthogonal grid, which provided the form to accommodate the co-operative and cosmopolitan ideas of Alexander the Great himself. In medieval Europe, the village street responded to the economy of agricultural labour by allowing each family a small plot of land for its own use, with the wider land beyond reserved for the feudal landlord. These needs created streets formed either by a connected row of houses with a kitchen garden behind (clearly expressed in the form of the Scottish burgh) or by a string of individual houses with strips of land beyond (as in the croft of Scotland or the Hufendorf of the German woodlands).

Thus the street became the most immediate and powerful physical expression of the values of our society. For us, society should not only protect individual freedom, but also offer the freedom to associate with others and to enjoy the unexpected encounter. Social encounters, whether planned or unplanned, allow an exchange of information that not only enriches our experience and knowledge, but provides a marketplace for cultural and commercial transactions. The street gives a recognisable form to public space, where potential purchasers can seek out products and services, and suppliers provide them. In the course of their transactions, the users of the street can acquire unexpected information – perhaps via a display of new products in a shop window, or a chance meeting with a friend. This is obviously true in a small town, but it should also be true in our larger towns and cities. Creating the spaces for people and for these encounters is fundamental to our vision for Plymouth.

In recent decades, the desire to pre-empt the possibility of conflict has been a key reason for the decline in the quality of the public realm and the street. Herein lies one of the great misunderstandings about the configuration of urban settlements. Conflict cannot be designed out, for the town or city street is only alive if it involves the potential for conflict. By providing the moments of choice between conflict and co-operation, the street can provide the basis of tolerance and become the major instrument of civilisation. To remove conflict, and consequently to deprive citizens of the opportunity to demonstrate tolerance, is to strike a death blow to the vitality of the street.

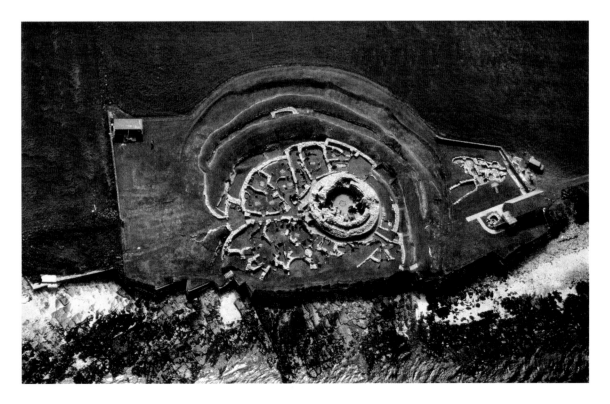

6. **Broch of Gurness, Orkney**
An early street system

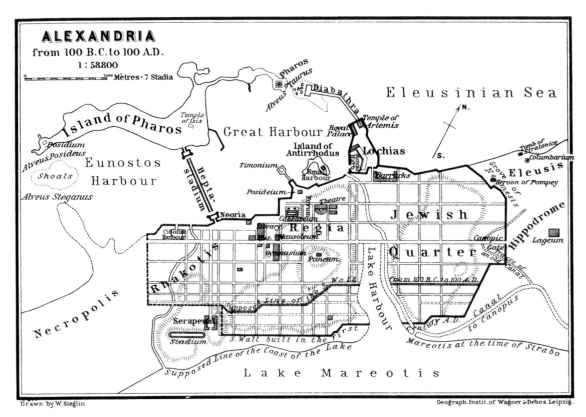

7. Alexandria
An early street grid of a culturally planned city

Behind the false idea of removing the inner conflict within the nature of our cities and our streets, lie two influential socio-urban theories that were developed in the last century. The nefarious influence of the first lingers with us today. It is founded on the belief that the city is evil and the country pure and good. It gave birth to the Garden City movement, an honest attempt to cure the social ills of an exploited working class by introducing the country into the city. On the one hand, the movement has left a legacy of urban countryside in the form of parks and botanical gardens; on the other, we have a suburban city form with streets that go nowhere. This is at odds with the vision of Patrick Abercrombie, who understood that one of the principal functions of the street is to connect. The broad street surrounded by railings that was designed to 'calm' the traffic by allowing cars to zoom through unhindered has extinguished this connecting function to such an extent that cities and neighbourhoods have become illegible.

The result – a package of problems that includes suburban sprawl, isolation of individuals and families, disintegration of formerly tight-knit communities, dependence on the motor car, division of territory according to socio-economic groupings, and social exclusion – has been a disaster.

The second theory emerged during the summer of 1933, when CIAM (Congrès Internationaux d'Architecture Moderne), a group of Modernist architects who had joined forces in 1928 to promote their ideas on town planning and rational design across Europe, held their fourth congress, on board the motor-yacht *Patris*. During the long August days spent sailing between Marseilles and Athens, they discussed the theme of 'The Functional City', and from this voyage of contemplation emerged a

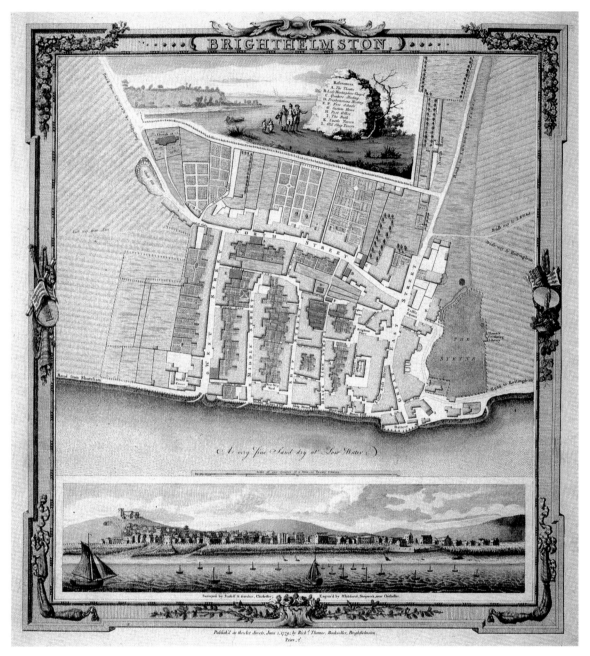

8. **Brighton**
The planned settlement of Brighton

document, forged into existence by Le Corbusier, that became known as the Athens Charter. It was to have an enormous impact, particularly through Articles 77 and 78, which sought to define the function of city planning. The first stated that 'the keys to town planning are to be found in the four functions: housing, work, recreation (during leisure) and traffic'. The second, that 'planning will determine the structure of each of the sectors assigned to the four key functions and will fix their respective locations within the whole'. Thus was born the abstract concept of the functional city. Concept was transferred into legislation in the brave new world of reconstruction in Europe after the havoc of war.

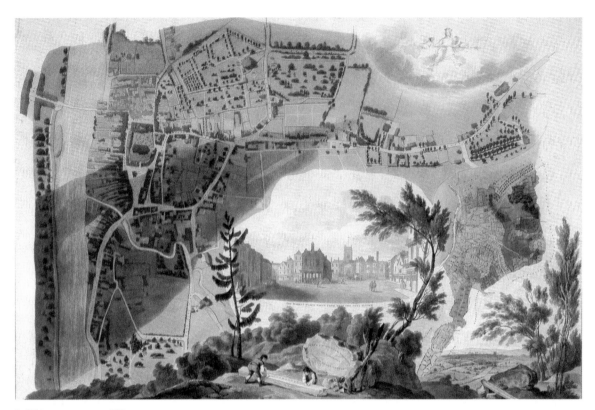

9. Kingston upon Thames
Planned through tradition, following an established code of practice and skills

The pernicious influence of the Athens Charter is due to the fact that these principles dovetailed so neatly with the interests of investors both public and private. The single-purpose building could be isolated from the difficulties of adjusting to the street or next-door neighbour, making design easy for the architect and engineer, construction easy for the builder and investment simpler for the financier. The functional city, constructed in a ring around the historic core of every European city, needed a separate functional solution for traffic. Streets were forgotten and replaced with a classifi-cation of traffic routes under the exclusive control of specialist engineers, who were responding to the needs of a consumer society obsessed with individual car ownership. When not in use, cars need storage and so the car-park made its appearance in the city. What an aberration – a park full of cars! The Americanism, 'the parking lot', is uglier, but much more accurate. It is time to change traffic routes back into streets and car-parks back into public spaces.

It is now generally accepted that the functional city is a fallacy, yet traces of this highly infectious intellectual virus remain to destroy the fabric of the street. The most virulent strain is the virus of segregation, which classifies streets into grades of traffic. The result is a city littered with the most absurd junctions and guard rails to control speed and protect pedestrians. Alternatively, streets are designated as pedestrian zones with no vehicles at all. The city responds to these stresses much as a living organism might, by mutating: segregated, pedestrian-only streets mutate into deserted and unfriendly pedestrian precincts, with shops that are closed and shuttered at night and empty properties above. Conversely, the restaurants and pubs along the streets that permit cars, buses and taxis, gather life. Such contrasting scenes can be found in cities across Europe, from Cardiff to Cologne.

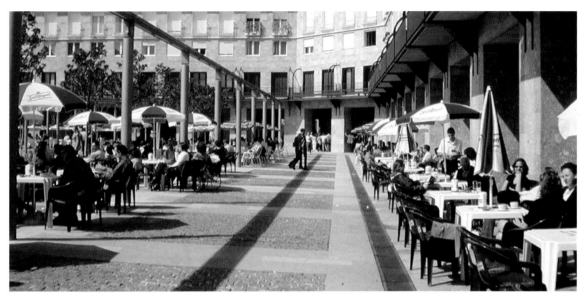

10. **Pamplona, Plaza Yamaguchi**
Buildings also define space

Pedestrians must be given priority in the city and there is a time and a place for them to take over, provided that two conditions are observed. The first is that pedestrian-only space should not be over-extensive (as it is, for example, in the historical centre of Krakow in Poland). Instead, it should act as an urban oasis, like Plaça de la Catedral in Barcelona, which is thronged with people at the intersection of intensively-used buildings and streets. Secondly, a street with traffic should always be within sight, thereby giving comfort and safety: to be on one's own in any pedestrian area at night can be quite threatening, but the glimpse of traffic on a nearby road restores calm by offering an escape.[3]

The scale of enclosure

The streets that we know and recognise exist not merely as two-dimensional plans, but also as the buildings that define the space and create the place. Every building forms part of the city to which it belongs: most blend together to form a general context, but there are others – public buildings such as schools and hospitals, or buildings in a striking architectural style – that stand out, like punctuation in a text. These landmarks allow one to pause and adjust one's perception of the city according to a different scale.

The character of the street is also determined by its topography – whether it is straight or curved, how wide it is – and the relationship of the buildings to the street (some with front gardens, some without). The more central urban streets have a richer morphology, or complexity of form. In Paris and Oslo, small courtyards that lead off the street give more depth to the building line and increase the space available for business or living activities. In London and Edinburgh there are mews, which accommodate a range of activities that supplement the major business and residential premises of the main streets. Then there are the larger central courts, like the hofs in Vienna, which contain community parks and may even contain schools – a feature found also in Dutch cities.

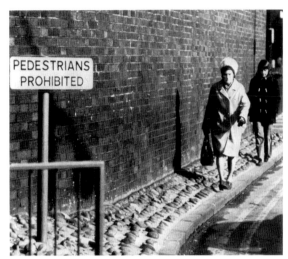 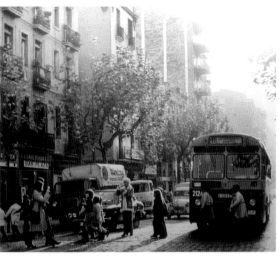

11. **Conflict**
The traffic engineer's response

12. **Acceptance of conflict**
The urban street

However, the corridor street is the more usual configuration of the urban character. This is a street that has a strong element of movement and flow, and leads from one particular place to another. Commerce is usually clustered where medieval trade routes once merged to form a marketplace, or where a deliberately designed square has been created, or where two streets run close to each other (for example, Southside Street and the Quay Road in the Barbican in Plymouth), where the stimulus of a short step to find alternative offers creates a dynamic relationship between the thorough-fares. The advent of the lift has allowed us to increase the activity (and economy) of the street with tall buildings. Such buildings can contribute to the scale of the enclosure, provided that they are both related to one another and linked to the corridor street nearer the ground. They need not be oppressive; in fact, they can create another kind of beauty, as in New York or Sydney, by introducing a welcome increase of scale that is appropriate to the city. This is essentially different to the isolated towers of the 1950s and 60s, such as those built in the Gorbals, Glasgow, or the claustrophobic constructions erected in the City of London during the planning free-for-all of the 1980s and 90s, which have caused the streets to lose their social role.

Therefore a fundamental objective in creating new urban structures and in renovating and improving old ones is to combine a discreet evolution of traditional elements with radically new architectural models. This objective is easily understood but difficult to bring about: nowadays the theory and practice of the most demanding kind of urban development revolves around this difficulty.

Movement through the public realm

One of the essential functions of the street is to provide a way of going from one place to another. For this reason places of destination are usually gathered alongside or related to the street system. The street therefore also becomes a place to be in, and in many ways the identity of the street is determined by the people who belong there. It is a shared space: the people who belong there share it with those who pass through on their way to somewhere else. Sharing creates conflicting interests, which have to be accommodated in the design and use of the space.

The social balance that the street demands can easily break down when one function is allowed to dominate. Too often, measures taken to manage the increase in car traffic have upset this balance by being too accommodating either to the pedestrian or to the motorist. The fear, and reality, of road accidents has too often led to drastic precautions that have destroyed the original functions of the street. Cities have been plagued by urban motorways interwoven with pedestrian over- and underpasses, or by mazes of streets that lead nowhere and are cluttered with strange forms to ensure slow driving. The street system has become a place of stress for both pedestrians and drivers, because each is demanding the same territory (the curious thing is that the pedestrian and the driver are often embodied in the same person assuming a different role at different times).

The answer is to accept that conflict is inherent in the city because it is these competing and alternating demands that make urban life the powerhouse of our civilisations. It provides not only the information that is sought but also the casual encounter of information that is not expected, the delight of discovery.

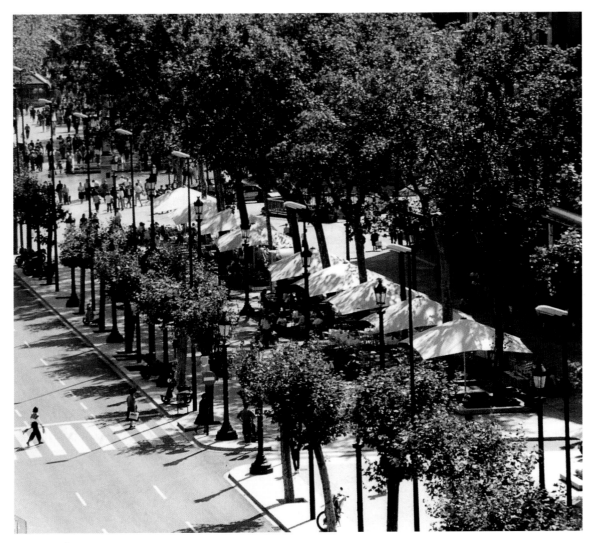

13. **Barcelona**
Movement through the public realm

To enable all these activities to function, the street system needs a recognisable structure. Perception of where one is and how to reach another part of the city relies on the existence of recognisable 'punctuation mark' structures at convenient intervals in the cityscape. These initiate a pause in movement or in perception of the environment, and could be something as simple as a change to double-height windows at ground-floor level, or a change in materials – something that the eye can grab to arouse interest and stimulation. A pedestrian needs such a structure within a maximum of 500 m, a driver roughly every 1,500 m.

In *The Image of the City*, Kevin Lynch makes a strong case for careful design (deliberate or accidental) to orientate movement through the city:

> A street is perceived, in fact as a thing that goes towards something. The path should support this perceptually by strong termini, and by a gradient or a directorial differenti-ation, so that it is given a sense of progression, and the opposite directions are unlike. A common gradient is that of ground slope, and one is regularly instructed to go 'up' or 'down' the street, but there are many others… Perhaps one can proceed by 'keeping the park on the left', or by moving 'toward the golden dome'.[4]

Seventy years before Lynch, Camillo Sitte understood the city as a series of perspec-tives, preferably enclosed spaces linked together. 'For [Sitte], the character of a town or a city lay in the public spaces that it could provide for its citizens, and its beauty lay in their rhythmic interrelationships.'[5]

The vision that we have prepared for Plymouth is not just three-dimensional, but incorporates the fourth dimension of time, experienced via movement through a sequence of spaces. Each of these spaces will be contained by the form of its surrounding buildings – both those that are already there and those that will be designed by other hands (with, we hope, a care that reflects the knowledge that they form part of the city). Even so, the city will have to live with its past, present and future errors – but then, that is simply a reflection of human fallibility.

The memory of place

There is a fifth dimension to every city: the collective memory of place. This is poignantly evident in the scene in Penelope Lively's novel, *City of the Mind*,[6] in which the hero drives down a London street and, upon seeing a blackened brick wall, vividly imagines the same houses blazing under incandescent clouds during the Blitz, the fire warden exhausted, and the hydrants running dry. The footprints of his childhood have been obliterated as the site has been rebuilt and occupied by later generations, reminding him how short our lives are compared to that of the city and its streets.

To retain the memory of place it is necessary, not to rebuild what was there in the past, but to draw on the past in order to rediscover the paths and footsteps of earlier generations. We should be guided as our predecessors were, by topography and the weather: the natural world changes little over vast periods of human activity, and therefore one can feel in the present the reasoning of decisions made in the past that suited previous cultures and material needs – such as, in Plymouth, the reasoning responsible for the location of the harbour.

14. **Plymouth**
Plymouth City Centre, post-war plan

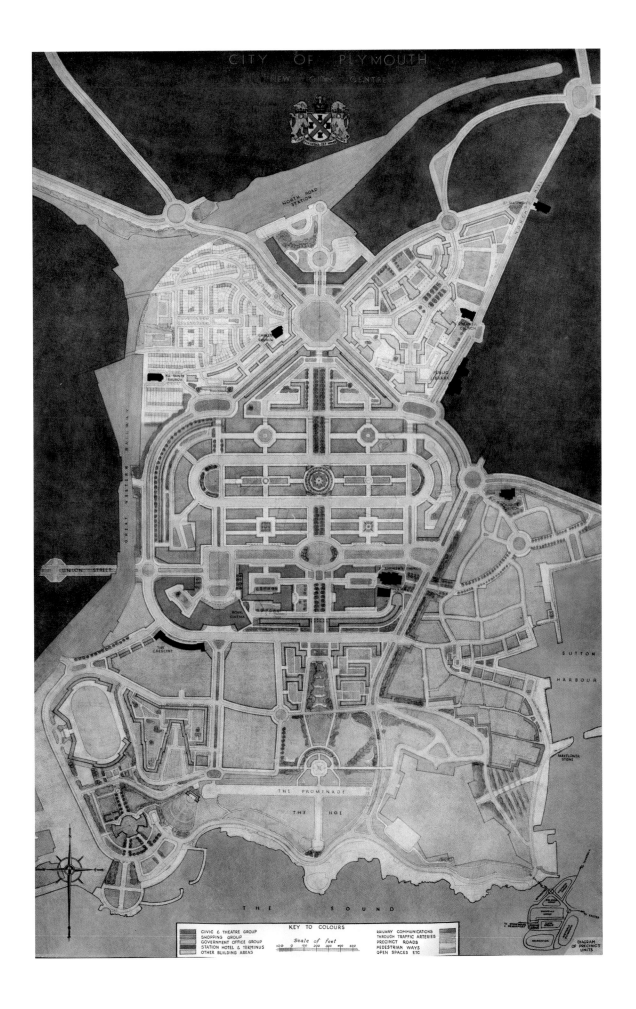

In renewing the city for the present and the future we must also create places that will strike new memories for the next generations. In order to do this we should understand Sitte's view, expounded in Vienna in 1889, of the city as a work of art:

> In order to realise this, city planning should not be merely a technical matter, but should in the truest and most elevated sense be an artistic enterprise … It is only in our mathematical century that the process of enlarging and laying out cities has become an almost purely technical concern. Therefore it seems important to remind ourselves once again that this attitude solves only one aspect of the problem, and that the other, the artistic aspect, is of at least equal importance.[7]

One could dismiss Sitte as a romantic, but his plea for considering the city as a work of art is continually repeated by critics and commentators, including Kevin Lynch, who writes from Massachusetts in 1959:

> A good environmental image gives its possessor an important sense of emotional security. He can establish an harmonious relationship between himself and the outside world. This is the obverse of the fear that comes with disorientation; it means that the sweet sense of home is strongest when home is not only familiar but distinctive as well.[8]

Our vision for Plymouth is also based on the belief that the city is a work of art carried out over generations, each one handing responsibility on to the next. It is also an essay in large-scale composition.

15. **Plymouth**
The Guildhall Tower. Familiar images give security of orientation

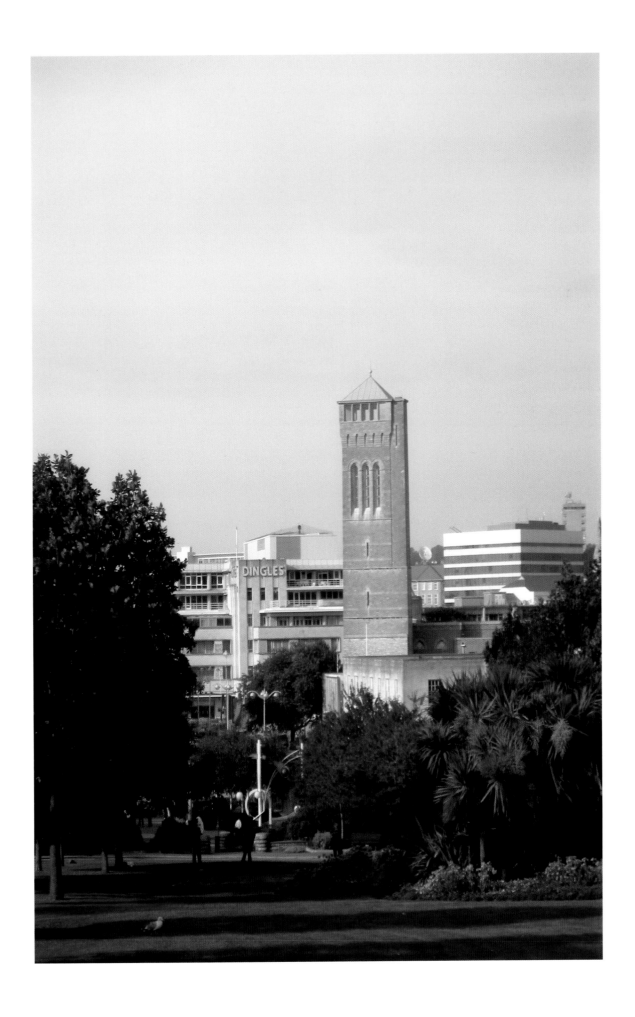

Notes

1. Sharp, T., *Town Planning*, Harmondsworth: Penguin Books, 1940, rev. edn. 1945. Sharp (b. 1901), a town planner who became senior research officer at the Ministry of Town and Country Planning, was the author of many seminal books on planning.

2. Paton Watson, J. and Abercrombie, P., *A Plan for Plymouth*, Plymouth: Underhill Ltd., 1943.

3. See Cullen, G., *Townscape*, London: Architectural Press, 1961.

4. Lynch, K., *The Image of the City*, Cambridge, Mass: MIT Press, 1960.

5. Sitte, C., *City Planning According to Artistic Principles*, transl. George and Christine Collins, London: Phaidon Press, 1965.

6. Lively, P., *City of the Mind*, London: Penguin Books, 1992.

7. Sitte, op. cit.

8. Lynch, op. cit.

Chapter Two
The Development Approach

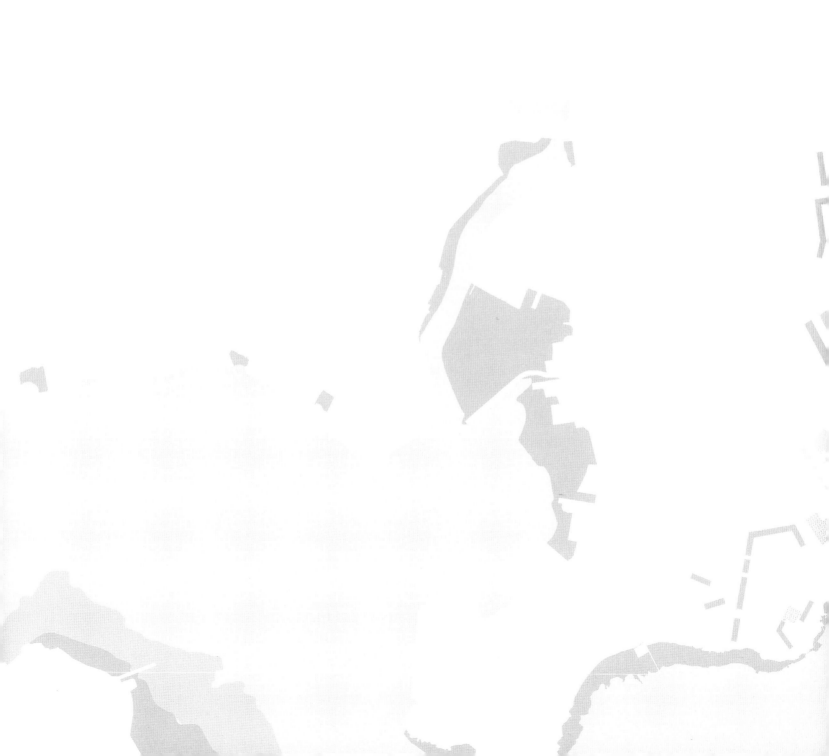

Chapter Two

The conditions

'After all, there's the sea, and green hillsides, and shops, and amusements; but there could've been so much more.'[1]

The historical form of the city

The fishermen who settled Plymouth in the eleventh century inhabited the area now known as the Barbican. They chose it for its sheltered position: a small natural inlet, it is tucked away from the prevailing westerly winds by the raised land of the Hoe. This physical asset of location – the deep, sheltered Sound, and the accompanying river mouths of the Tamar and the Plym – provided the opportunity for the maritime and military-led growth of the city through the following centuries.

The significance of the waterfront in the process of urbanisation is that it fuelled pockets of growth at the points where there is access to deep water. The building, slipping and repairing of ships in adjacent berths resulted in the tripartite development of Devonport, Stonehouse and Plymouth. Whilst the three towns were largely independent, each with its own living, working, and retail areas, the rapid pace of economic growth in the eighteenth and nineteenth centuries drove expansion inland at such pace that by 1914 the towns were officially agglomerated into one urban area – Plymouth. This process of inward growth and development produced an urban form that physically linked the new heart of the city back to its waterfront origins. Both the connection of the urban form and the localised sustainability of the three centres are clear in plans showing the city before the Second World War.

Following widespread destruction of the central core of Plymouth during the war, the Beaux-Arts plan on which the reconstruction of the city was based reversed much of this historical relationship with the waterfront, focusing greater attention on the two new axes of Royal Parade and Armada Way, and the system of vehicle circulation around the core. Abercrombie's desire for 'an inner ring road enclosing the shopping and business area of the city' was fully achieved in the implementation of the plan.

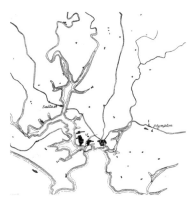

16. **1800**
The three urban communities: Plymouth, Stonehouse and Devonport

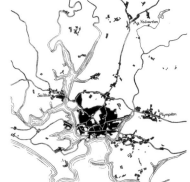

17. **1939**
The compact city begins to expand

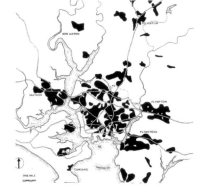

18. **1960**
The fragmented city, with suburban satellites

The single use imposed by the reconstruction and the subsequent resistance to change endemic among commercial landlords (who are, after all, only responding to the realities of institutional investment) contributes another level to the physical isolation, ensuring that the activity of the City Centre is focused on retailing, to the detriment of any other uses.

In its pursuit of mono-functional use, therefore, Plymouth has turned its back on history and in the process it has lost the human scale of connection between its heart and limbs. Our vision seeks to reunite the City Centre with its extensive waterfront, active harbours, and the landscape beyond.

Population

According to the census of 2001, the City of Plymouth currently has a population of about 240,000. This is 10,500 fewer persons than were recorded living there in 1991. Remarkably, the population has grown relatively little since the beginning of the twentieth century, when the figure was 211,000.

It is fair to report that the income levels of the population are lower than those of neighbouring Exeter, and this is due to both the time distance from London (3 hours by train rather than 2 hours for Exeter) and the historical reliance on the shipbuilding and repair industries dominated by the military client base. Exeter has benefited from a more diverse economy built upon the service sector.

As a regional centre Plymouth also supports a wider 'travel to work' area, bringing the total employment catchment to approximately 350,000. From a retail perspective the catchment area is reported as almost 500,000, yet movement in from rural areas also drives the move of businesses to out-of-town locations, which are seen as more accessible by car than the City Centre.

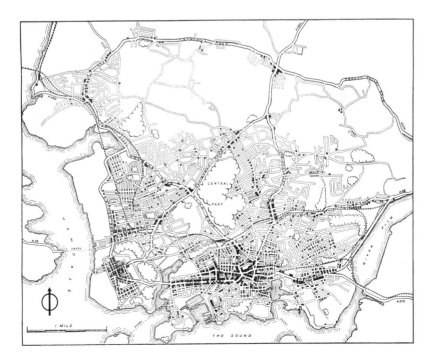

19. Plymouth
The pre-war structure, with shops marked in black

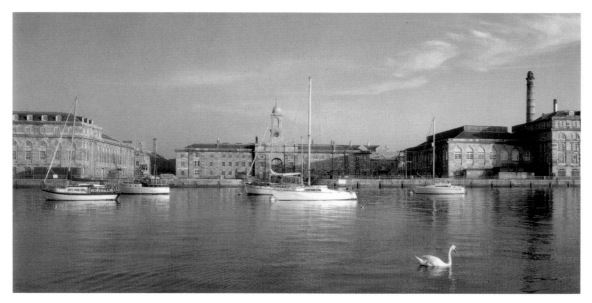

20. Royal William Yard, Plymouth
A high-quality urban redevelopment by Urban Splash

The impact of the retail-dominated core of Plymouth is reflected clearly in the way in which the population is spread throughout the city. The distribution of the population across wards varies greatly, with one of the lowest population densities (27 p/ha) found in Sutton ward, which covers much of the City Centre. Much higher densities, of up to 70 p/ha, can be seen in the wards immediately surrounding the City Centre, in the strongly-established communities of Mount Gould, Drake, and Stoke.

Over the past decade, the South West region has experienced significant in-migration of economically actively people looking for better quality of life, as well as those of retirement age. Conversely, the region is a net exporter of 16–24-year-olds, thereby losing much of its youth investment to other parts of the country. This process has been particularly marked in Plymouth, where the number of people aged between 20 and 24 declined by 31% between 1991 and 2001. Among 25–29-year-olds, the decline for the same period was 35%. The shrinking of the youth population illustrates wider concerns that Plymouth is not performing the role of an economically sustainable city. In essence, Plymouth seems to fall far short of the potential offer for lifestyle, workplace and urban attractions that such a uniquely positioned and naturally endowed waterside city should be able to provide to a waiting population. In an age of electronic communication, changes in work patterns have reduced the need to commute every day, permitting new migrants to the city to retain a work connection with London and the South East. The quality of life and natural environment that Plymouth offers provide the opportunity for new waves of population migration to increase its urban population substantially over the next 20 years. Such are the pressure on space and the cost of living in the South East, that estimates of 100,000 additional population 'escaping' to Plymouth over the next 20 years do not seem unreasonable.

Creating a city with a population of between 300,000 and 350,000 is one aspect of our vision.

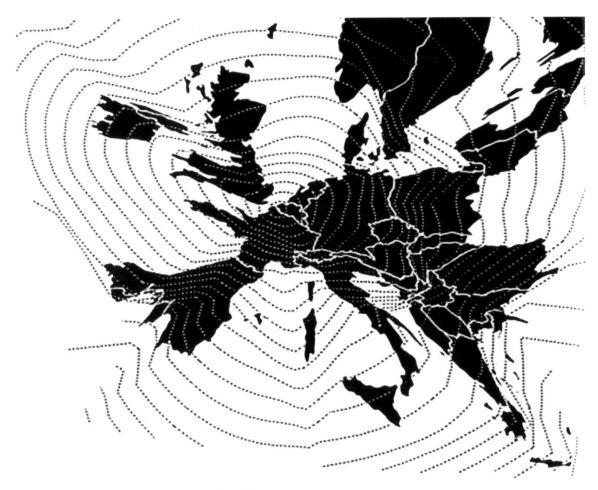

21. Europe transformed (Rem Koolhaas)
The impact of the TGV link to Lille – infrastructure generates new geographies of time and space

Transport

The city is located on the border of the Devon and Cornwall peninsula, and is served by the dual carriageway A38 'Devon Expressway', which connects to the M5 at Exeter and continues onwards to Bristol, Birmingham, South Wales and London. Despite the distance the city is clearly connected both to the North, the South East and the South West, with strategic routes providing set journey time connections to Bristol of 1.5–2 hours, and to London of 3–4 hours.

Plymouth Airport provides hub connection to London, but limited service to Europe when compared to other UK city airports. The existing airport located within the city is constrained in the long term by the length of the runway. Within the broader European context there exists a macro-urban structure of cities that enjoy the economic benefits of an efficient air travel network. The second-tier cities of Rotterdam, Frankfurt, Lille and Genoa all have airports and good connections. Throughout our discussions in connection with this study, we have continually reinforced the importance of an airport connection within this network, to enable Plymouth to take its place in the hierarchy of European cities.

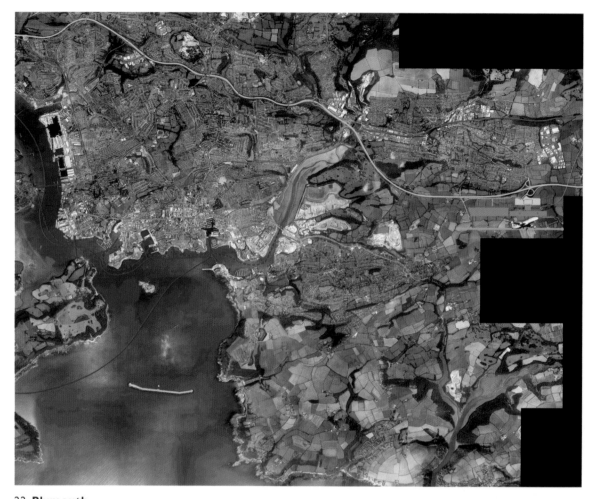

22. Plymouth
Major transport connections: road, rail, Light Rapid Transport (LRT), sea and an unresolved future for the airport

The centre of the city is the magnet for bus and coach services that serve both outlying suburbs of the city and towns throughout Devon and Cornwall. This service reinforces the importance of the city as a centre for health, education, retailing and leisure. The tradition of public transport use by the existing population of the city provides relatively high passenger numbers.

To support the strategy of reducing car dependence within the centre of the city, the development of high-quality bus services leading to the introduction of a framework of fixed link tram or light rail is an essential infrastructure investment. This supports the vision objectives of reinforcement of the City Centre and development of its capacity for both residential and business accommodation, and the infrastructure will permit the new areas of development at Millbay, Devonport and Royal William Yard to flourish. Without such investment, the city will continue to rely on the private car, and bear the associated impact on quality of life, public space, and poor pedestrian movement.

Property

In line with national trends, the residential property market in Plymouth has consistently surged in recent years. Significantly, recent developments in the waterfront areas of the city have reached record values for Plymouth, and demonstrate the appetite at the higher end of the market for high-quality and contemporary urban living accommodation. The development of Royal William Yard by Urban Splash epitomises the opportunities that are available, and continued provision of this type of accommodation is an essential component in the process of attracting high-quality business investment.

However, the nature of the post-war reconstruction of the City Centre as a predominantly retail estate has largely precluded opportunities for living within the very heart of Plymouth. The impact of this historic zoning is clearly evident in the streets of the City Centre: devoid of any leisure or service functions, they are empty and quiet outside shopping hours. The proximity of the University of Plymouth and the demand for student accommodation has prompted the residential conversion of a small number of buildings within the Abercrombie footprint, but there is still much unused capacity within the upper floors of many retail units. The Draft Local Plan[2] addresses this issue with provision for mixed-use development on three major sites, but the key task is to find a typology of development and public space that generates sufficient high-quality, desirable living space to meet demand and to challenge the established perception that Plymouth is 'grey and dirty'.

It is unfortunate that developers and the City Council have tended in the past to propose and permit development of the poorest acceptable quality. This has perpetuated a run-down feel to the City Centre and reinforced the view that secondary accommodation (i.e. for students or for budget hotels) is the only option for the City Centre. The problem is exacerbated by the development of stunning, award-winning buildings in fringe locations, such as the Theatre Royal Workshops outside the City Centre. This lack of confidence in the City Centre has no doubt influenced decisions to invest elsewhere.

Retail

Within the post-war City Centre Plymouth contains around 1.4 million sq ft of retail floorspace, much of which is within pedestrianised areas. This volume of retail space secures Plymouth's position as a sub-regional shopping centre, and many major stores are represented, including Dingles (House of Fraser), Derrys, Marks & Spencer and Debenhams. The prime retail area is centred around New George Street, although the quality of the retail offer declines notably as one moves north. Although vacancy rates are reasonably low, it is evident that space within the retail core of the city is underused, and this is confirmed in the Urban Capacity Study published by the City Council.[3]

One of the key impacts of the volume of retail floorspace has been the provision of car parking on a large scale in the City Centre. The perceived isolation of the City Centre from the surrounding areas of the city appears to fuel the reliance on private vehicles.

Office

Plymouth plays a major role as a service centre for the far South West region, with the service sector accounting for the largest percentage of employment in the city.[4] Financial services, health, public administration and education are the largest sub-sectors. Recent growth in the bio-medical and research and development markets has been attributed to the quality of life that Plymouth can offer, and these markets will be crucial to sustaining future growth.

Office provision is largely in the area immediately surrounding the City Centre shopping precinct, although recent commercial development has focused on the out-of-town business park locations. In town, rental levels have increased over the last 18 months, from £8 to £10 per sq ft, whilst out-of-town rents are higher, at around £12 per sq ft. Providing the right conditions and opportunities for occupiers to choose the City Centre rather than out-of-town locations will be a key element in the process of regenerating the heart of the city. Discussions now taking place with major employers – such as the Department for Work and Pensions, which at the time of writing is looking to occupy 80,000 sq ft adjacent to the Civic Centre – appear to be having positive results. Attention should also be given to attracting smaller businesses to occupy components of mixed-use developments.

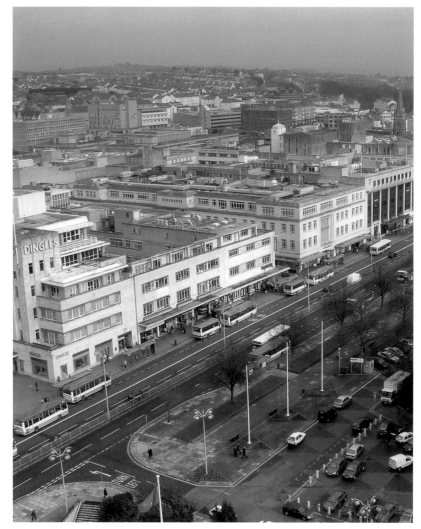

23. **Plymouth**
Royal Parade, marking the edge of the retail island

Leisure and tourism

Plymouth currently acts as a destination for mostly short-stay tourists, who are often attracted to the city as an excursion from longer-stay trips in the region. The tourist offer in Plymouth is based on heritage and history, shopping, leisure attractions such as the National Marine Aquarium, and opportunities to visit peripheral sites such as Mount Edgcumbe Country Park. The National Marine Aquarium attracts the largest visitor numbers in the city, with 425,000 visitors in 2002.

Current trends in the tourism industry towards greater demand for high-quality, short-term breaks with increasing emphasis on the natural environment, place Plymouth in a strong position to improve and market its credentials as an outstandingly well-situated city. Realising this opportunity, through the development of the waterfront and the enhancement of the relationship between the waterfront and the city, is placed at the heart of the MBM strategy.

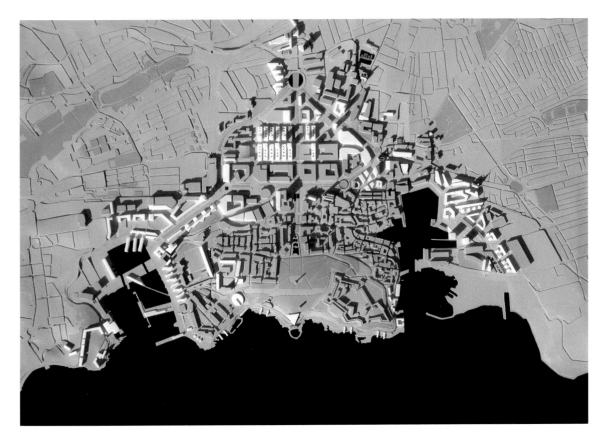

24. **Plymouth**
Proposed new structure connecting the City Centre with the waterfront

The opportunity

In our opinion there is a direct correlation between the possibilities that the historic form of the City Centre has created and a new future programme of intensification and diversification.

Plymouth enjoys an enviable position to embark on such a programme, as the city has an unusual degree of control over much of the land required for transformation. The redevelopment in the 1950s and 1960s that was based on the 1943 Plan was carried out following the traditional leasing structure for town centres. The City Council retained the freehold, and granted building leases to developers, who in turn constructed and let the accommodation on rack rents. The resulting properties were subsequently sold as investments to institutions, which remain as largely passive investors in receipt of the rental income. The recent CB Hillier Parker review of the City Centre identifies approximately 13 head lessors.[5]

The freehold that the City Council retains over the 90-acre (36-hectare) site at the heart of the city is the key component that will permit its transformation. This heartland site – laid out on an exemplary grid, with buildings now 50 years old, predominantly for shopping and retail, and with only a handful of investors controlling its future – is a 'strength for the city' and a key opportunity for renewal.

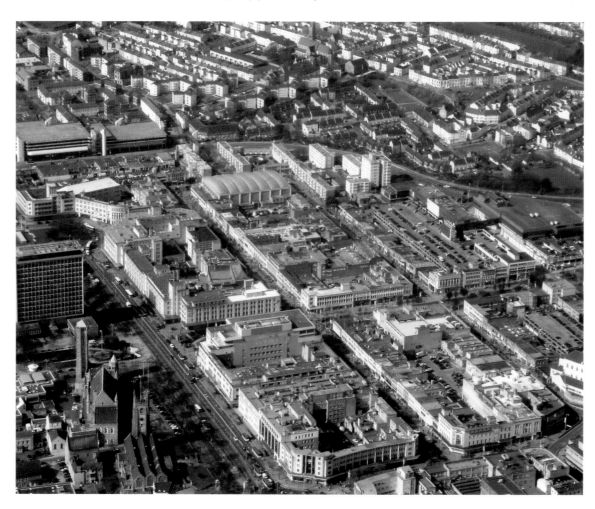

25. Plymouth
The City Centre retail island

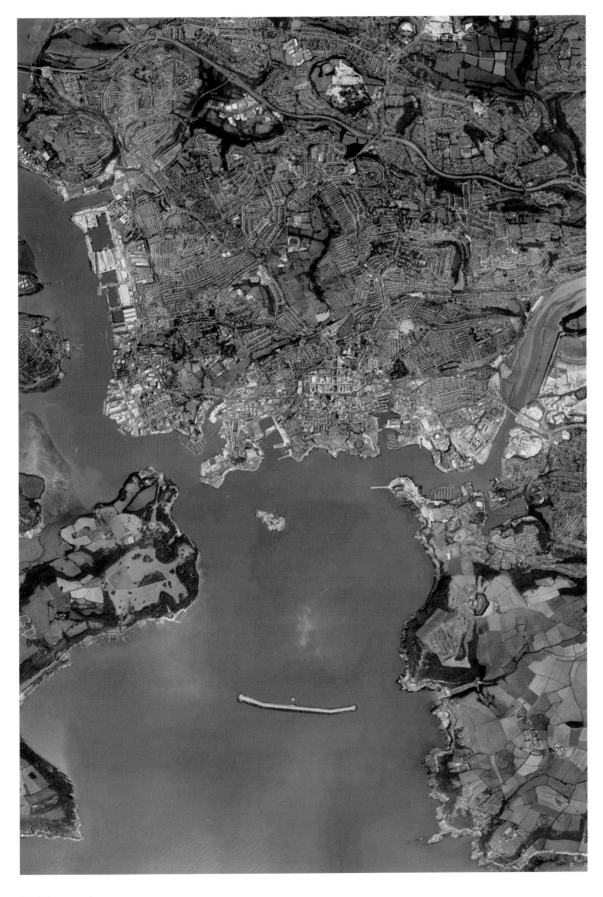

26. Plymouth
City of green and blue – a natural setting second to none

39

Plymouth has the huge advantages of its waterfront location, and should follow the example of other cities, such as Liverpool, Newcastle, Barcelona, Genoa and London Docklands, that have supported inward investment to take advantage of the unique environments generated by their respective waterfronts. Plymouth has begun this process with the waterfront developments at Sutton Harbour, the Royal William Yard development and other developments on the Hoe.

The catchment area extending into Devon to the east and Cornwall to the west, consists of small settlements where demand for housing far outstrips supply, and this has pushed up property prices. The environmental constraints on expansion and limited infrastructures of these small settlements ensure that supply is ultimately constrained and prices continue to rise. The demand in these areas, driven by an expanding population of locals, weekenders and retired folk, underlines the potential for the high-quality urban alternative of the City Centre. It needs to be developed with a style and imagination that is missing from the current approach. Plymouth, as a principal urban area of the region, must positively capture this demand and thrive upon it.

Our vision looks forward 20 years with this ambition in mind, and the development assumptions follow that timeframe.

We see the potential for a transformation of the City Centre on a par with the regeneration that has taken place in northern cities such as Glasgow, Manchester, Liverpool, Newcastle and Leeds. Twenty years ago, these cities' centres were deserted, with large, derelict warehouses and former industrial sites awaiting refurbishment. Imaginative leadership has rejuvenated these areas, with mixed-use schemes of inner-city accommodation, bars, studios, offices and galleries. These places have rekindled the excitement of living at the heart of the city.

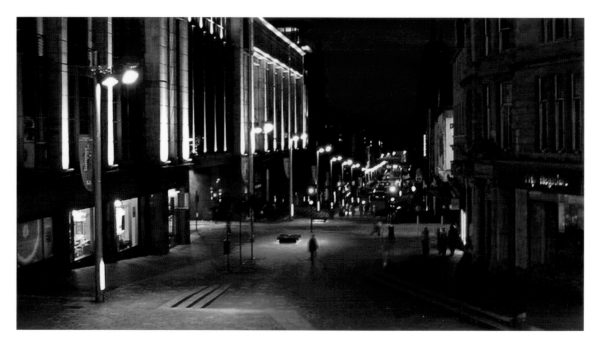

27. **Glasgow**
Buchanan Street regeneration

Within the City of Plymouth a similar opportunity exists, but in this case the requirement is more for redevelopment at densities that support and invigorate the urban context. This calls for imagination and a quality of architecture and place-making that can encourage the population to migrate inwards to live in the City Centre.

We see an opportunity for a more dense development of mid-rise buildings and occasional towers positioned within the Abercrombie grid. It is an opportunity for high-rise living that is unique to the UK's historic cities, offering views out across the city to the waterfront, exploiting the natural topography of the valleys that lead down to the Barbican and out to Millbay. We see this as an opportunity to create a 'mini Manhattan' of the South West, consisting of residential towers, mixed use, retail, restaurants, bars, and offices.

Lifting spirits, raising expectations, and demanding the best architecture, design and development that will respect and respond imaginatively to the opportunity and potential that is offered by this unique waterside city, will ensure that within the 20-year term of the vision, Plymouth takes its rightful place among the other European cities of equal size.

42

Notes

1. Nairn, I., *Britain's Changing Towns*, London: BBC, 1967.
2. Plymouth City Council, *City of Plymouth Local Plan*, First Deposit Draft, 2001.
3. Llewelyn Davies, *Plymouth Urban Capacity Study*, 2001.
4. Office for National Statistics, Census 2001.
5. CB Hillier Parker, 2000.

Chapter Three
The MBM Vision for Plymouth

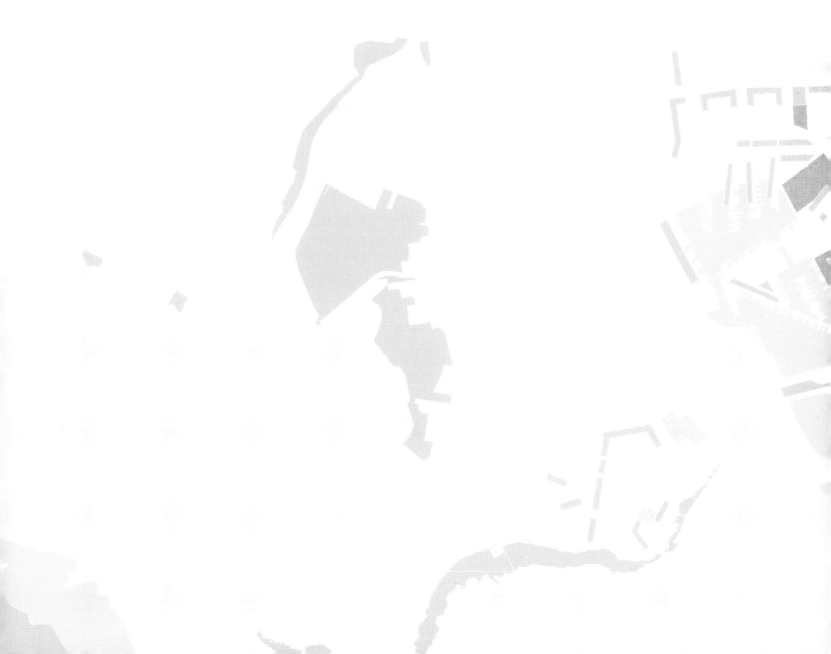

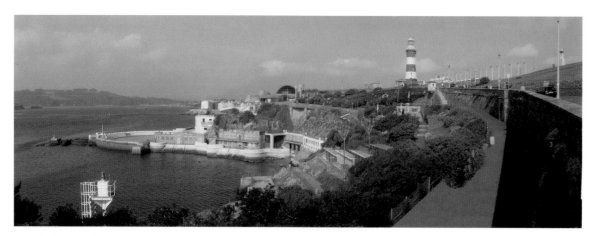

28. The Waterfront
Tinside Lido, projecting into the sea, has a pivotal role at the centre of the Hoe

Recovery of the waterfront city

Plymouth has one of most enviable locations of any city in the world. The views across the waters of the Sound and the rolling green hills to the east and west provide a setting of outstanding natural beauty. Few cities have the opportunity to establish a close relationship with a surrounding landscape of such high quality.

The waterfront has long been the leading element of this landscape. It could be described as the frontage to the landscape and façade to the city. It has provided for the industrial and military economy that fuelled the growth of the city, and has more recently transformed much of this heritage into a major tourist offer. In marketing terms, the waterfront is Plymouth's Unique Selling Point. All the recent high-value, premium residential sales within the urban area have been on the waterfront. The busy calendar of water-based events and demand for moorings in the city's marinas show that demand for leisure facilities continues to grow. The waterfront also plays a significant role in the economy of the sub-region, maintaining activities from operational ports to marine science research, even as the traditional local, water-based industries decline.

The city waterfront is currently defined by a number of attractions – buildings, events and spaces that each draw and recreate their own activity. In areas where such attractions cluster, such as Sutton Harbour, the result is a lively and dynamic mixed-use 'quarter', which becomes a recognisable and self-sustainable piece of the city. Other 'pieces' of the waterfront – the recent development of Royal William Yard, the refurbishment of Tinside Lido, the Mount Batten Centre, the Theatre Royal Workshops – present their own story; yet the picture is somehow not complete, and there is no one element that holds the waterfront together. The challenge at the city scale, and therefore the challenge for this vision, is to look beyond the 'quarter' and propose a spatial strategy through which the existing fragments and the future opportunities of the whole waterfront can achieve a critical mass that both defines and drives the vitality of the City Centre.

We envisage the waterfront of Plymouth as an arc – a curved spine of activity loosely flowing east-west and drawing the influence of the water back into the city. Our repair of the city form is based on this leading structural element of the city, and our vision is guided by three underlying principles: movement, attraction and relationship.

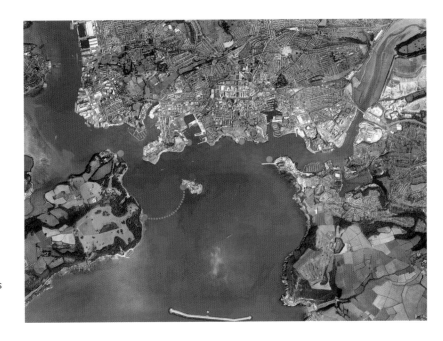

29. The Sound
The city waterfront forms part of an arc within the green hillsides, and provides many opportunities for potential landing points

Movement: transport at the waterfront

The waterfront is historically a place of movement and transport. From the departure of the *Mayflower* in 1620, to the current ferry operations serving mainland Europe, Plymouth embodies the atmosphere of both embarking on adventure and of destination and arrival. For many European visitors, Plymouth's waterfront may be the first and last piece of Great Britain that they see.

This strategic gateway function of the waterfront must be enhanced through the provision of improved port infrastructure as part of the development process at Millbay. Providing the facilities to support cruise ships and the vital input they can bring to the local economy needs to be balanced with meeting the demand for high-value residential properties on the waterside. Locating such facilities at Millbay could bring vital energy to the area, and help to balance the activity of the more established and successful Sutton Harbour.

But movement is not simply about arriving and departing on long journeys. It is more often a journey from home to work, from work to shop and eat or drink, or a trip for recreational or social arrangements. Many such trips could be accommodated by an improved water transport service, which could not only reduce road-based movement, but would also provide a vital passenger base to a water service that could also target tourist requirements. We have taken recommendations from the marine transport study[1] and used them to identify potential landing points for a new and improved water transport service.

The waterfront should also be a promenade for pleasure and delight where people can simply walk or cycle between events and attractions, and this requires commitment to the public realm. From the strategic South West Coast Path to local connections such as the route from the Hoe to Millbay, the form of development and the definition of the public space are crucial to enabling and encouraging people to enjoy the city on foot.

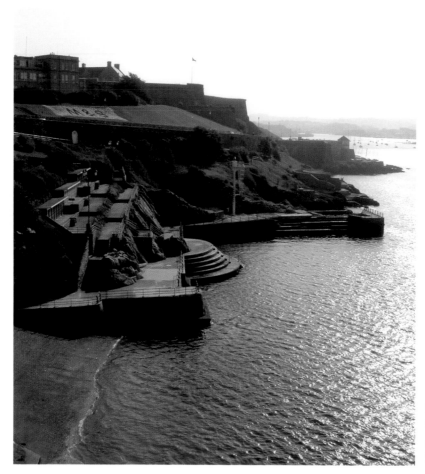

30. The Waterfront
Where all citizens can stroll
and observe the activity of
the Sound

Attraction: a waterfront for all citizens

If Plymouth is to succeed in drawing its own citizens and others from further afield to experience and enjoy the waterfront, then there must be sufficient activities and attractions to satisfy the urban explorer.

Many successful attractions exist on the waterfront. The National Marine Aquarium is Plymouth's top attraction, with nearly half a million visitors in 2002. Our vision is to develop this tourist offer (and we offer proposals to exploit two major opportunities), but also to give equal importance the smaller-scale attractions (events, spaces, viewing points, moments) that define the unique character of Plymouth.

We see much of the opportunity for an improved tourist offer between Millbay and Sutton Harbour, and for this reason we have made recommendations for the Hoe foreshore. The process of regenerating Millbay will not only create a series of vibrant places, but, crucially for the city, will provide a new dynamic between the two harbours, placing new emphasis and demand on the area between them, and completing the urban 'circuit'.

For those who wish to venture further afield, to Royal William Yard, Devonport, or Mount Edgcumbe, the water transport system in itself should prove an attraction.

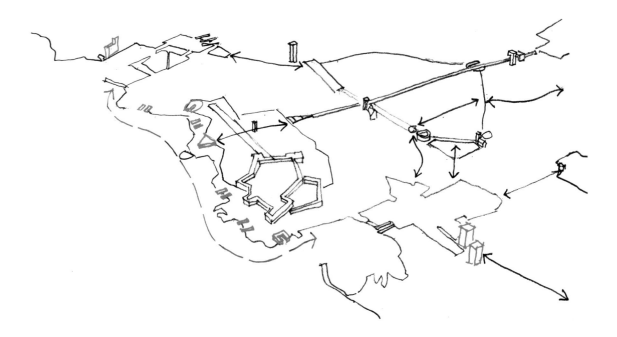

31. Concept
The Hoe waterfront as a link between Sutton Harbour and Millbay

Relationship: the waterfront and the City Centre

As the premium location in the city, the waterfront has a responsibility to take the lead in the process of change. Attracting new residents, businesses, and tourists requires a supply of high-quality buildings and spaces.

But the waterfront, and the premium for living, working, and playing that it holds, belong to the public realm, not the private. If the waterfront is to channel positive change back into the city, close attention must be given to the form of the streets and buildings, and the nature of the uses contained within them. In historic locations such as Plymouth, the key to this relationship of inclusion can often be found in the urban forms that were generated from a different set of cultural, social, and economic values, and it is to these lost forms that we can look for guidance.

In summary, the City of Plymouth benefits from an extraordinary waterside setting that compares with other waterside cities throughout the UK and Europe. Comparable cities have used their setting and their architecture to establish their credibility on a world stage (for example, Genoa the European City of Culture 2004, and Liverpool the European City of Culture 2008). It is for Plymouth to build upon the MBM vision to establish itself within the same firmament.

Invigorating the Abercrombie Plan

Many people may find it strange that Plymouth City Centre is thought to lack an urban atmosphere. On most afternoons, and especially on a Thursday or a Saturday in fine weather, it presents a lively crowd of shoppers strolling from side to side and street to street, with some places so full that one can hardly move. So what is meant by 'an urban atmosphere', and why is it desirable?

The answer is simple. The plan of Watson and Abercrombie called for multi-storey buildings enclosing the wide streets on an appropriate scale, which would have given proper weather protection and provided upper floors for other uses. They planned frequent north-south links to make it easy to go from one street to another. The interiors of the blocks were for service access to the shops, but were also laid out with gardens. In other words, the 1943 plan for Plymouth sought to create an urban atmosphere through variety. Alas, it was not carried through as planned. The buildings are too low and the blocks too long, so that the streets now have a windswept, suburban appearance. In the classic 1960s pop song, *Downtown*, Petula Clark celebrates the many opportunities to meet people and discover things that one can enjoy by going downtown. A city the size of Plymouth deserves a downtown for everyone, not just one age group. Our vision for the City Centre is to make it a real downtown, and not just a successful open-air shopping centre. It needs to offer residents and visitors a 24-hour life, with restaurants, pubs, specialised shops, a choice of entertainment and culture. It must have quiet places, but enough activity (with buses, taxis, cars, etc.) to make it feel safe.

Watson and Abercrombie's plan for the City Centre was a masterpiece of modern English town planning. It must be conserved, not as a fossil but in an invigorated form that responds to present circumstances and shifts in cultural values. In other words, we must identify its soft or weak parts, where we can act, and readjust to balance the poles of attraction where people will want to go. Our response to this opportunity should not be constrained by protectionist policies: the nature of the grid structure must be respected, but the plots can be rebuilt to a greater density, and new cross-streets can provide the permeability that Watson and Abercrombie originally wanted for the City Centre.

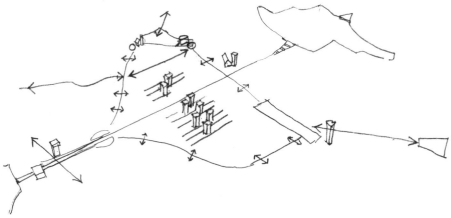

32. **Concept**
A connected and diversified city centre

Our vision creates a released, connected, diversified and defined City Centre.

A released City Centre

Plymouth City Centre is freed from its triangular traffic collar, allowing the economic, social and cultural energies to circulate through the body of the city. Western Approach, Cobourg Street, Charles Street, and Royal Parade become avenues with central pedestrian or green strips, and pedestrian crossings at surface level. Car parking facilities are removed from the centre of the city blocks, and resited at the edges, where existing facilities are underused.

A connected City Centre

Redevelopment of large sites around the edge of the City Centre allows new buildings and spaces to recover lost relationships with surrounding neighbourhoods. Movement across the City Centre is improved, with cars and pedestrians sharing the horizontal streets at all but the busiest shopping hours. The original purpose of Armada Way – to form a grand vista linking the train station to the Hoe – is recovered through a simplified landscape design, with movement enhanced by the introduction of a public transport link.

A diversified City Centre

Comprehensive redevelopment of the blocks on either side of Cornwall Street provides a new focus: a 'living street' of intensity defined by a series of tall buildings, with lanes of living, working, leisure and retail space to the north and south. The finer grain of building provides increased retail frontage on a human scale, with flexibility for office and residential accommodation above.

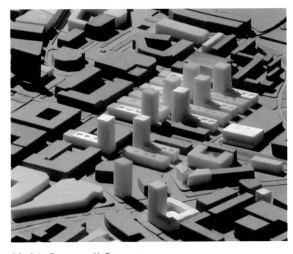 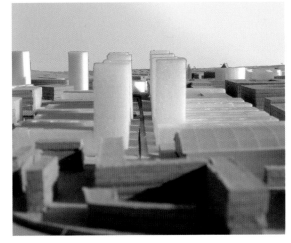

33, 34. **Cornwall Street**
A new 'living street' with side lanes and lookout towers

A defined City Centre

Above all, the City Centre is no longer defined by its isolation and retail use. Instead, it is defined by varied architecture that exploits the rigidity of the grid, with tall buildings providing stunning views of the city and water, grand gateways from both water and land, and a wide range of visitors, including weekend tourists who come to enjoy the rich history and culture of Plymouth in the City Centre, as well as along the waterfront walks.

Note

1. Scott Wilson, *Plymouth Sound and Estuaries Water Transportation Study*, 2003.

Chapter Four
The Elements of the Plan

Millbay

The historic harbour of Millbay has been identified in our study as one of the greatest opportunities for transformation, and thus a key contributor to the future success of Plymouth. It is an area of complex interactions between the port (which has particular operating requirements), the adjacent military base in the impressive Stonehouse Barracks, and the City Council and other parties interested in strategic level mixed-use development of the area.

We have proposed an infrastructure and development strategy that will transform Millbay and create a new magnet for urban regeneration to support the economic development of the south-west corner of the City Centre. In the context of our broader Plymouth strategy, Millbay epitomises the lost relationship between the City Centre and the waterfront, and is therefore an important locus for change. Our comprehensive approach to shaping the form of this territory between the waterfront and the City Centre has been informed by the Area Regeneration Strategy completed by Lacey Hickie Caley Architects,[1] and the policies outlined in the Draft Local Plan.

Beneath the tempting simplicity of this 'clean slate' waterfront site exists a series of challenges and constraints that have influenced and shaped our response. Firstly, there is the question of access to the port, and the large volume of traffic it generates. The roadway wrapping around the inner basin precludes a meaningful relationship between the water and the area to the north. Furthermore, the military occupation of land to the west of the harbour both constrains the connection to Stonehouse Peninsula, and restricts the development potential of the glorious grain silos, a true cathedral of industry. Our vision for the future challenges this position beyond the present, and looks forward to the possibility of recovering parcels of military land to the benefit of the wider community. The work currently under way in Devonport illustrates the potential of such a recovery to rebuild and strengthen connections within the community. Similarly, to the east of Millbay, it will be essential to form meaningful connections and interactions with the existing, established neighbourhood of West Hoe, in order to avoid creating more 'exclusive' – and socially divisive – enclaves of the kind produced by previous waterside developments.

In essence, to capture the opportunity for the city, the regeneration of Millbay must respect and relate to the city as a whole, and not solely to the opportunity for waterfront development.

The proposal

In order to secure this opportunity for the city, our plan proposes a new vehicle access route to the port, to be located along the existing Battery Street axis and passing beneath Millbay Road to the harbour. Improving the relationship with the development sites to the north, this route will also allow a public transport corridor to feed into the heart of Millbay, and provide traffic options that can relieve pressure on the north-east connection to the city. It is a balancing act that respects the need for the Union Street area to be connected to (and perceived from) the water, something that must be achieved by channelling activity, as well as improving legibility.

The two-way relationship between Millbay and the City Centre, the result of geography and industrial history, has largely been eroded. We see the repair of Millbay and the

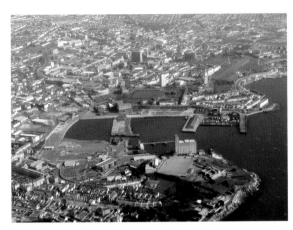 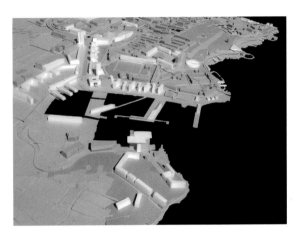

35, 36. **Millbay**
Millbay is the western counterpart to the more easterly Sutton Harbour

repair of the City Centre as two interrelated processes that require the creation of a new link that is both legible and multi-modal. Following the axis of the existing Bath Street, we propose to achieve this connection with a boulevard that begins at Derry's Cross and flows towards the water, following the topography that originally served to drain the City Centre, and later took the railway connection to the dock. Marked at its entrance and northern corner with a tall building, the procession for the pedestrian down to the harbour marks a clear and legible departure from the character of the City Centre, and an invitation to movement beyond. The suggested form along the boulevard is of four or five storeys, with opportunities for taller elements within it to mark the progress of the route, and provide accommodation with views across the waterfront. Some of the existing buildings along the route are of good quality and historic interest; further detailed studies should identify which of these may be retained and incorporated within the courtyards and grain of the new form.

The second connection to the City Centre is achieved through the recovery of the historic route of Millbay Road, lost within the current arrangement of buildings at Derry's Cross that were designed as part of the Abercrombie plan. This route, marked by views of the Civic Centre and the Clock Tower, incorporates many minor pieces of character (such as the cluster of trees adjacent to the Ballard Centre), and reveals the beauty of the Crescent and the Duke of Cornwall Hotel along its path. The imminent redevelopment of sites at Derry's Cross provides an opportunity for the city to recover this piece of historical linkage in the near future.

The success of this new neighbourhood for the city will rely heavily on encouraging the sense of waterfront place. As at Sutton Harbour, this character of place will require investment and engineering. The inner basin, if it were provided with a lock to retain the high water level, could provide a marina with an additional canal through the Glasgow Wharf leading to the triangular piece of water by the East Quay, where there would be space for 250 moorings. This would provide an attractive and active addition to the series of public spaces along the quays. People are not attracted by water or public space alone; it is the range and diversity of the activities that take place there, the characters involved in them, and other characters observing the same that make these pieces of the city attractive and enjoyable.

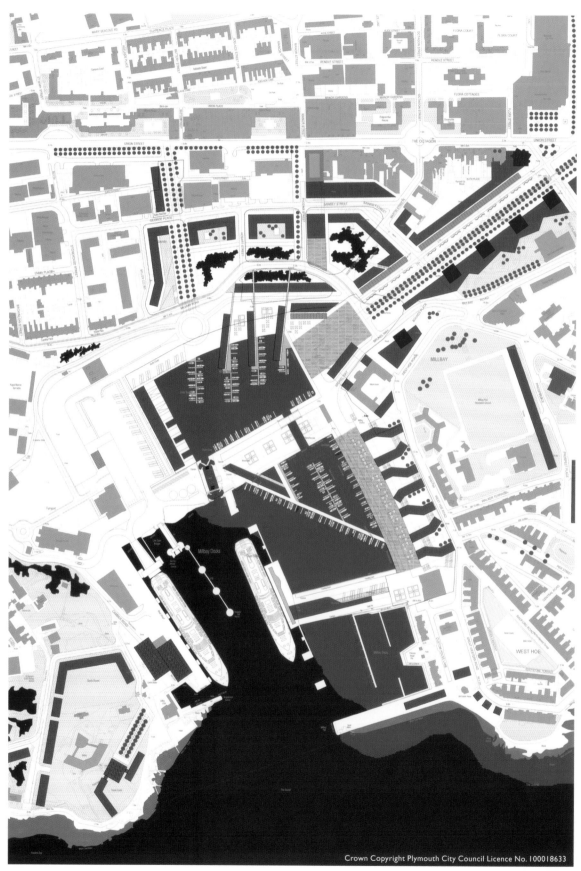

37. Millbay
Proposed forms of redevelopment indicated in red

Moving to the harbour edge, our plan has incorporated the existing proposal for a marine industry facility (of approximately 4,000 sq m) adjacent to the port area of the inner basin, which is welcomed not only for economic reasons and the vessel activity that such a facility should bring, but also as a visual 'buffer' to the port operation and parking beyond. Careful consideration of the views from the eastern side of the harbour across to Royal William Yard and Mount Edgcumbe beyond will be required in the progression of this building, and the facility should therefore avoid the typical 'shed' image through consideration of its fifth façade (the roof). Marinas also require a wealth of more open structures that together animate and structure waterside spaces, and elements such as dry docks and repair yards should all be carefully considered within the design, as too often the tendency to hide industrial practices takes away the very essence and character of place. This is the essence that Gordon Cullen refers to as the 'busy industrial scene permanently *en fête*'.[2] Also in the inner basin, our plan explores a typology of 'finger' blocks, feeding down from the upper level of Millbay Road, that echo the traditional slipways and pier structures of dockside installations, and provide both physical and visual connection to the Union Street neighbourhood to the north. These 'fingers' or piers should contain residential accommodation over two or three storeys lifted above the quay and inner basin on stilts, with an undercarriage at quay level for commerce, restaurants, etc. and preserving views of the harbour and Drake's Island from the development behind.

At the intersection of the new boulevard and the inner basin we have shown a public space of city-wide significance, defined sufficiently by surrounding buildings with active ground-floor uses. Every city requires a space like this to house special temporary events, both cultural and commercial. It is not for us at this stage to propose designs for such a space, but we feel it will be important to preserve elements of the rich industrial heritage of the location within the materials and form of the public space design.

The northern development

Beyond Millbay Road to the North, we propose a series of U-shaped buildings set within, and fronted to the south by landscaped gardens. These would accommodate housing with communal gardens and swimming pools facing the strip of pocket public parks and views across the Sound.

We support the proposal, put forward by a local community group with a keen interest in music, to create a large auditorium at the old Palace Theatre (now known as the Academy) in Union Street. On the north side of Sawrey Street, studios and workshops could accommodate facilities for teaching, rehearsing, recording and other activities associated with the performing arts. Immediately south of the Palace Theatre and forming part of the U-shaped urban buildings, there could be a new concert hall with a public space facing the harbour for outside events.

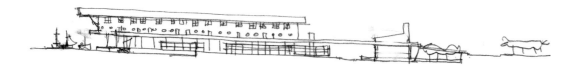

38. Millbay
The proposed slipway lofts in the inner basin

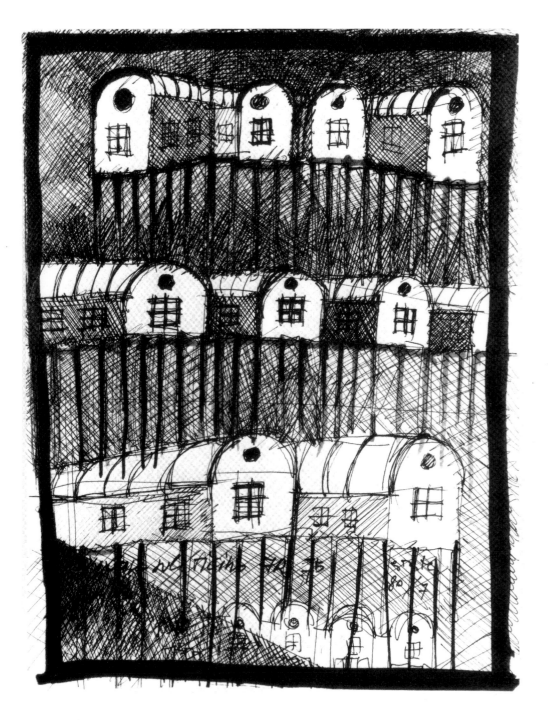

39. Concept
Sketch by Aldo Rossi

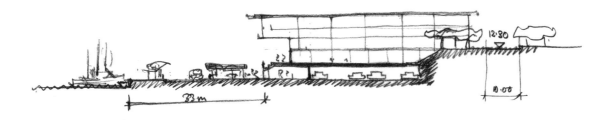

EAST WHARF.

HOE ROAD
MILLBAY.

40. **Millbay**
Proposed deck and filter dwellings on the East Quay

The east side and the piers

The core residential element of Millbay, we propose, will be represented by a series of housing blocks arranged roughly perpendicular to the water, allowing through-connections to the existing neighbourhood of West Hoe, and providing the stimulus for future redevelopment of the nearby Territorial Army site. These blocks are shaped to afford wide distribution and variety of views, and would incorporate the sectional change in level, rising from perhaps four floors above podium level, to two storeys at the Hoe Road façade. Substantial parking would be accommodated under the podium of the development, making use of the height differential, and could be accessed from West Hoe Road. At ground level on the waterside, these buildings would accommodate bars and restaurants, with outdoor seating areas on the dockside similar to those in the Olympic Port in Barcelona, or at Somerset House in London. This would facilitate the connection between the Hoe and Millbay.

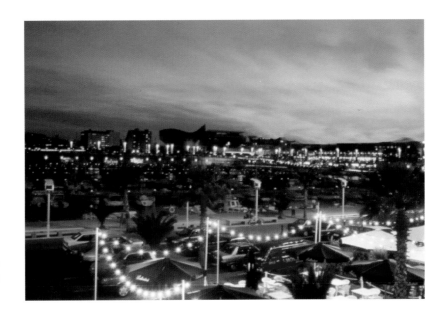

41. **Olympic Port, Barcelona**
Using a similar section for the East Quay would provide facilities for restaurants, bars and a car-park

The shallow and tidal nature of the middle basin led to suggestions that it could be filled in to provide more development space, but we see the supply of marina space as crucial to the image and success of the development. Millbay has the gift of a unique waterside setting, and to reduce this would be to deny the whole city an opportunity for the future. We propose a retaining wall and a system of locks, which could provide an adequate depth to allow medium-sized craft into the marina. The inner pier should provide public access, and could house leisure facilities such as a sailing club, or other marine uses. This is particularly important as Trinity Pier is a terminal for cruise ships, and therefore functions largely as a private space.

Moving seaward, we suggest limiting the development of Millbay pier to the eastern end, in order to preserve views from the wider Millbay area to the sea. The vision is to build upon a harbour in a waterfront setting; to enclose that setting with ill-considered buildings or to infill the water area would be to destroy the very nature of the place, and lose the essence of the opportunity.

The western side

On the western headland of Millbay, we envisage the opportunity to make use of the famous grain silos as the basis for an international conference centre, which would be built alongside and above the existing structure. Spectacular views of Drake's Island and the Sound would make it one of Britain's most prestigious conference venues. Nearby and on the Eastern King Point, a five-star hotel set in landscaped grounds would complement the conference centre. Clearly, this will not be achievable until such time as the military no longer require the site, and detailed studies for vehicular access and parking will be necessary, as will careful analysis of the nature of the connection to Royal William Yard.

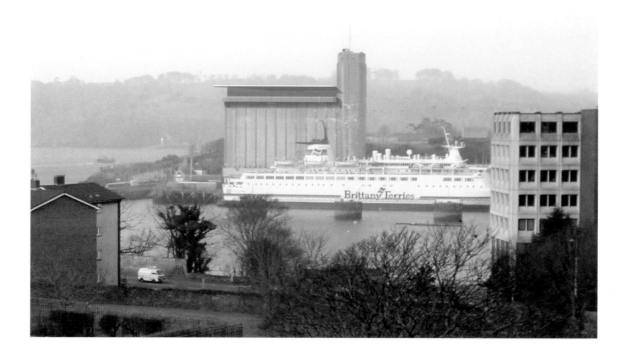

42. **Millbay silos**
This prominent feature could be an anchor for a new conference centre

The development process and impact – recommendations

Implementation of the proposals outlined here will need to be led by the construction of the infrastructure necessary to support the development framework. Primarily, the infrastructure would generate the access down Bath Street, relieve port traffic, and improve the setting to the dock – in all creating a clear connection to the City Centre and a setting for inward development. Meeting the cost of the acquisition and infra-structure works will require funding from the development opportunities of sites within the Millbay area.

The proposed delivery mechanism would be a series of site and development partner-ships commensurate with the scale of the ambition, but these development partnerships can only come about when the development agency has invested in the infrastructure and regenerated the public realm. This process configures the roads, public spaces and car-parks, identifies the sites and defines the quality and capacity of the individual building blocks that make up the proposed masterplan. Current conditions generate high values and high demand for residential accommodation, but this development vision is based upon a mixed-use form of development that will include restaurants, bars and shopping, as well as car parking and office accommodation. It cannot be left to market forces.

From our analysis of the office market in Plymouth we consider that Millbay provides the 'lifestyle' opportunities that could help foster the market for creative businesses, and to some extent offer an alternative to the office parks at the edge of town. Reviewing the success of Sutton Harbour, it is clear that very little office accommo-dation has been created there. Our vision embraces the long-term sustainability of the Millbay area by recognising the necessity of providing a full range of uses. In particular a 'critical mass' of business space will ensure that the redeveloped area can provide employment opportunities for the long-term regeneration of the area.

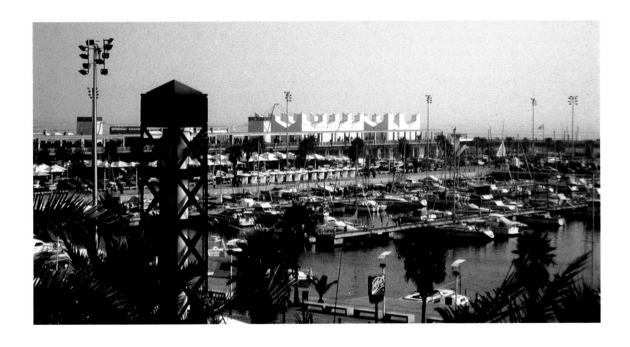

43. Olympic Port, Barcelona
A 'wet square' with a marina could be the new aspect of Millbay

The mechanism for delivering the commercial space, integrated as it is in the overall proposed development envelopes, could take the form of a revenue/capital split in the development outputs. Analysis of the east side development, where uses are predominantly residential, together with the public space at the south-east corner of the dock, suggests how such an approach might work. Where these uses are more commercial the development theory would be to use development partners to construct the infrastructure of the whole, with cost contribution from the public sector to fund the infrastructure. Capital returns from the completed residential sales would fund the construction of the entire mixed-use development, with the public sector retaining the income-producing/commercial elements and encouraging through subsidised rents the gradual occupation of the commercial elements. The strategy is founded upon creating a supply of commercial space before the demand for it actually exists, funding it from the demand for the residential accommodation. If commercial space can be supplied in attractive and well-designed buildings with flexible sub-divisions, small companies may begin to move in; these pioneers generate a buzz that encourages larger companies to occupy the remaining office space.

The MBM vision will thus be delivered through a consistent mixed-use strategy, and by the development of a critical early core which generates a sense of place and sets down the blueprint for further future development matched to the demand profile that will become a reality following the success of the first stage. It is worth noting that the launch of the Urban Splash development in Royal William Yard attracted some 3,000 visitors in the first weekend, which gives some indication of the demand for high-quality residential accommodation within the city.

The South West of England Regional Development Agency (SWERDA),[3] English Partnerships (EP)[4] and the City Council are in the process of commissioning an Action Plan that will develop a 'clear and optimal framework' for development of Millbay. To assist that process we recommend that consultants consider the following issues that need further work to take forward the MBM vision to the next stage:

- Identify additional land holding and ownership and identify costs and constraints associated with it for periphery and linking areas encompassed within the vision

- Identify the development plots and decide on the phasing of their development

- Review the delivery approach outlined within the vision and estimate costs of infrastructure works and associated car parking, and commercial accommodation in a first phase

- Prepare outline proposals for development of parcels that accord with the principles of the MBM vision

- Estimate the market sales generated by elements of the development

- Determine the public sector funding requirement needed to allow the private sector partners to deliver the first phase.

44. **Olympic Port, Barcelona**
Bringing an urban context to the marina

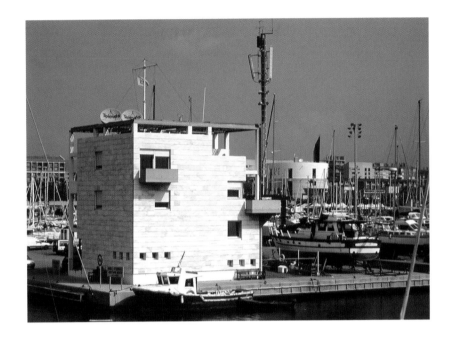

The City Centre

Two quotes, separated by 50 years of experience, illustrate the change in attitudes across a generation of city authors. The first, from the 1943 *Plan for Plymouth*, forms part of Watson and Abercrombie's explanation of their new road layout: 'The east limb of the ring road is planned to pass eastward of Old Town Street… forming a "cut-off" from Historic Plymouth'.[5] The second is a recent expert panel's verdict on Abercrombie's vision:

> Time has judged the concept itself to have been far from perfect, so beguiling on the coloured plans but so disappointing on the ground… Why do the buildings themselves, save along Royal Parade, seem too thinly spread and too small in scale to create a sense of true urbanism?[6]

Post-war planning and what we now understand to be good urbanism are different in many ways. Abercrombie did a fine job of giving a physical form to the theories of his age. However, as discussed in Chapter Two, the search for rational order in his post-war rebuilding of Plymouth is now widely recognised as the culprit that eroded the very essence of urbanism. It is a reassuring start to the process of change to have this constraint recognised in the Local Plan, and potential solutions explored further through the City Centre Urban Design Framework.[7] Our approach meshes carefully with these two key documents, as it is both strategic in its assessment of the role of the central area as an essential component of the City, and it is spatial and local in its recommendations for shaping new forms and spaces to address recognised problems.

45 (Overleaf). **Proposals for the City Centre**

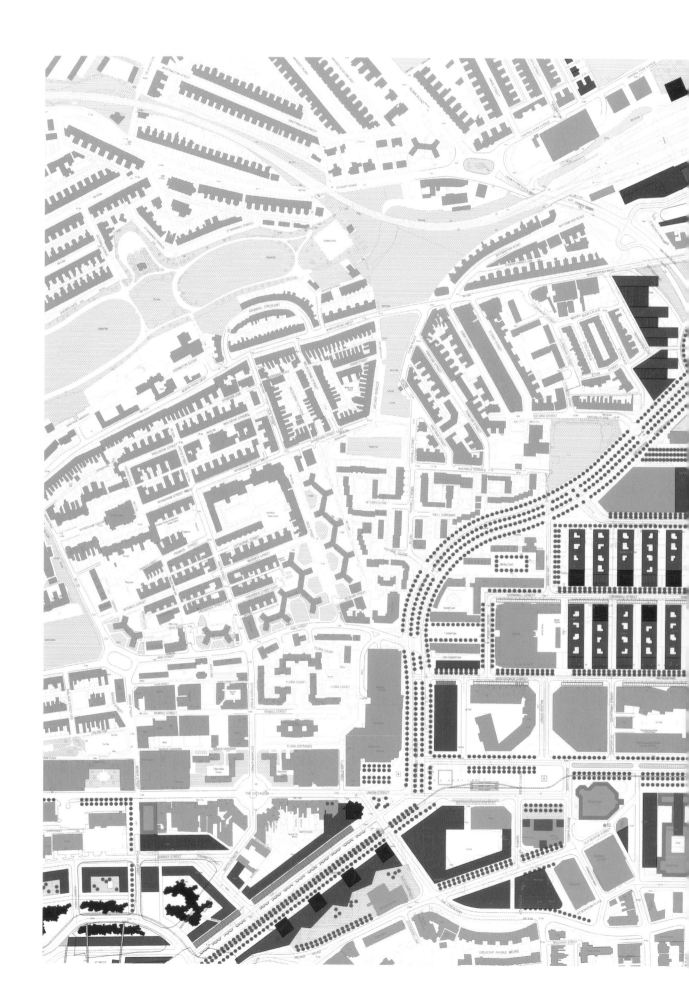

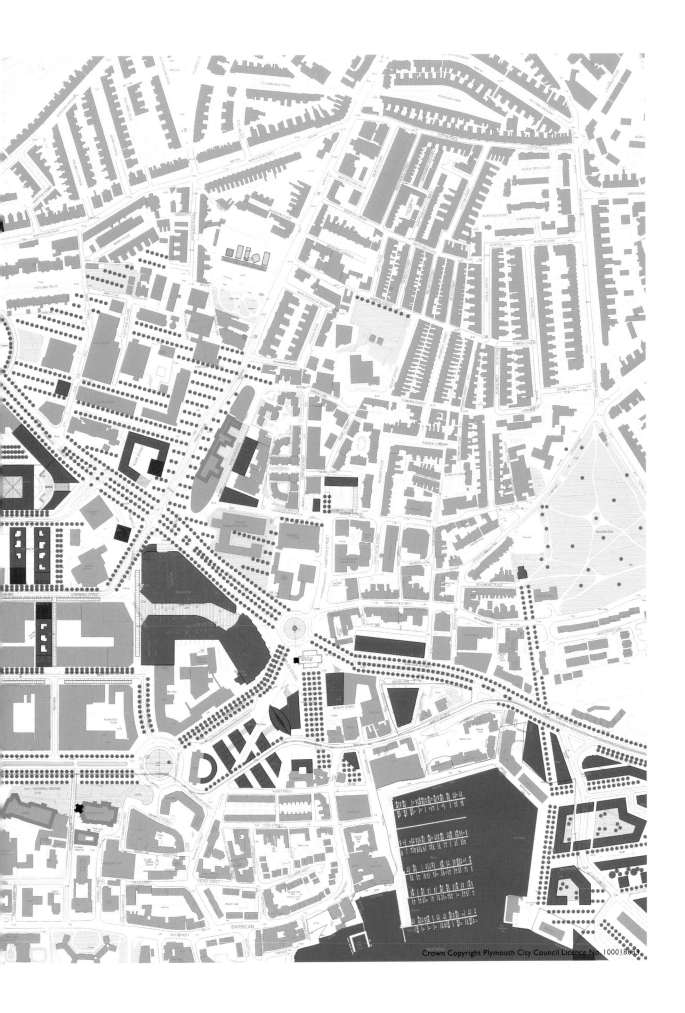

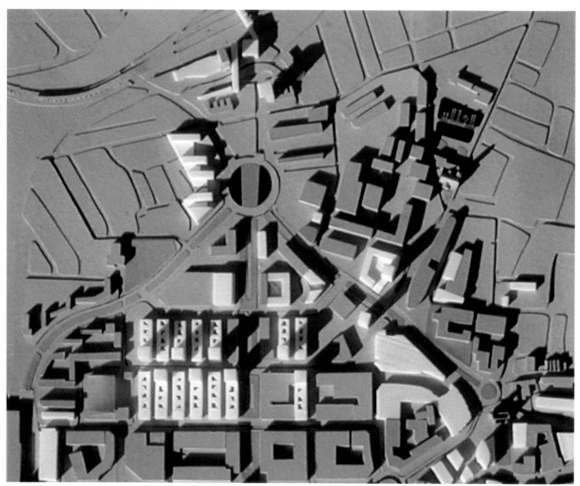

46. City Centre
Model showing proposals for the heart of the city

Indeed, our work in the City Centre takes its brief largely from the City Centre Urban Design Concept Plan and Urban Design Principles within the Local Plan, and presents a development and public realm strategy to explore the realisation of these concepts. Achieving our vision of a real 'downtown' is led by the following policies:

■ Reducing the impact of the ring road on pedestrians and users of the City Centre

■ Repairing and remaking connections with all the surrounding areas

■ Positive creation of a mix of land uses within the City Centre to create a more vibrant and sustainable centre

■ Improving movement within the central area and through to the adjacent areas.

The heart of the city – an exploration of intensity

The transition in quality of the built environment is clearly visible as one moves south through the City Centre. As commented upon in the opening quote, whereas Royal Parade succeeds in delivering the high quality architecture and environment envisaged in Abercrombie's plan, much of the area to the north is of low quality, and of a density, use and form that fails to provide a sense of urbanism.

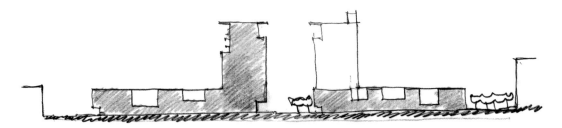

47. **Cornwall Street**
Proposed new living quarter

As it contains a collection of buildings now more than half a century old, many of them due for replacement or redevelopment, the central area presents a series of opportunities for the scale of intervention required. Our project here begins by taking the two large blocks allocated for comprehensive redevelopment between Mayflower Street and New George Street (west side), where we propose a fundamental reworking of the building morphology within, and respecting, the historic grid. The form of the Abercrombie superblock with its perimeter development of shopping and its service yard to the rear is transformed with a series of north-south routes running between New George Street, Mayflower Street and Cornwall Street. These routes are based upon a grid dimension of 20 m for the development and 10 m for the width of the road, representing an adjustment to a new, more intimate, scale. The building frontages are arranged in alternating strips providing a route for servicing, car parking, rear entrances to upper parts and mews-style offices/studios, alternated with extension of the shopping frontage through to the cross-streets. Beyond the logic of an exercise in urban form, this subdivision will both increase footfall and 'Zone A' frontages — the prime floor area at the front of a shop, which has a substantially higher rental value than the rear — to the economic benefit of the occupants.

The form of the development, based upon a four- or five-storey terrace on frontages approximately 10 m wide, will provide flexible elements of accommodation, robust enough to sustain changes in demand and programme. We envisage residential use on the upper floors, with retail and business functions on the lower floors. This is a new grain of development for the City Centre that aims to provide a level of intricacy and freedom of movement that has been lost in the realisation of Abercrombie's plan, and the many years of layering upon it.

Defining this new city neighbourhood within the visual cityscape, and exploiting the opportunity for intensity, a series of tall buildings is suggested, to be located along Cornwall Street. Primarily residential, these would provide stunning views across the city to the sea in the distance. Where poor-quality buildings exist on the eastern side of Armada Way, it is proposed to consider the extension of this model, providing a 'living strip' of mixed-use activity from Frankfurt Gate in the west, through to the University in the east.

At the northern end of Armada Way we have suggested, for consideration, the establishment of two cultural buildings that will mark the entrance to the city, working alongside the proposal for the cultural quarter around the University on North Hill.

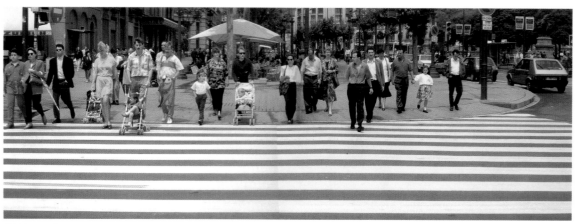

48. **Barcelona**
Balancing the priorities to give pedestrians their space

The edges of the City Centre

Within our strategy, the two southern corners of the City Centre precinct – as the gateways from both east and west and the key connecting points with the waterfront – require specific attention to their form.

Derry's Cross

Recent commercial developments at Derry's Cross have reinforced the function of this area as a culture and leisure focus, yet it remains largely impermeable from the south, and has a poor relationship with Millbay and the older hotels marking Millbay Road. Our structure here is founded upon the re-establishment of the historic route of Millbay Road, curving through the site toward the City Centre, and enclosed on either side by block-defining buildings.

As the land slopes down to the north, the opportunity for placing car parking underneath development here is clear. Emerging proposals for the development of the Civic Centre car-park site contribute to this vision of Derry's Cross as a lively area for working, leisure, and culture.

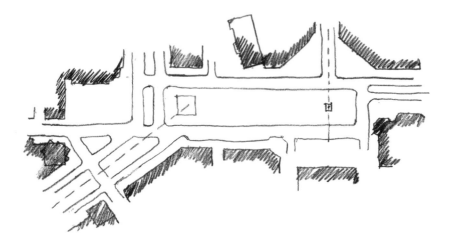

49. **New Derry's Cross**
The connection point between Union Street, Millbay, and the City Centre

To define the heart of this western end of Royal Parade, we propose a civic square, marking the significance of the interface between Union Street and the City Centre, and the new neighbourhood of Millbay to the south, and providing adequate space for possible Light Rapid Transport (LRT) and bus interchange. Proposals for the redevelopment of Colin Campbell Court are emerging as we produce this document, and should respond to the challenge of addressing the ring road in a more urban manner.

Bretonside

Bretonside, on the south-eastern edge of the City Centre, presents a poorer urban environment than its counterpart at Derry's Cross, directly hindering the relationship with Sutton Harbour. This part of the city represents more than just the approach to Sutton Harbour, as it is also a key entrance point to the City. Yet here at the threshold of the centre, we find Charles Cross Church, the memorial to those citizens who died in the Second World War, now disgracefully abandoned and downgraded to the realm of the highway. Although it still stands proud on the skyline of the city, its role as a landmark is sadly undermined by the reality of its isolation on the ground.

Re-routeing the A374 to release Charles Cross Church and providing a pedestrian link that effectively offers it back to the people of Plymouth are the first steps towards recovering a sense of place in this lost location.

The current commercial interest in the redevelopment of Bretonside makes the task of carefully planning how it should relate to the rest of the city all the more urgent. Our plan for this area reduces traffic along Exeter Street to two lanes, converting this elevated structure into a more public place, which would filter down into the Barbican alongside rows of stepped buildings, perpendicular to Exeter Street.

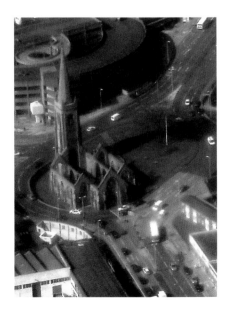 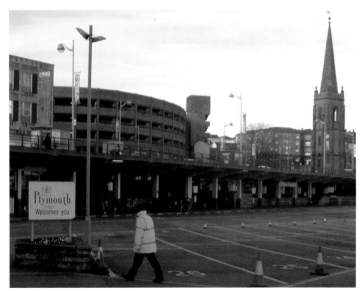

50, 51. **Charles Church and Bretonside**
Charles Church should function as the gateway to Sutton Harbour. Bretonside Bus Station also forms a barrier that disrupts links to the water

We envisage relocating the functions of the bus and coach station to a new integrated transport hub at the railway station. It is important that decision on this element in the plan be given priority in the emerging proposals for Bretonside, as the additional development opportunity created by releasing the bus and coach station site can contribute to the costs of this relocation.

The form of our proposals for the Bretonside site ensure cohesion and legibility between the University area, the proposed P&O shopping mall, and the bustling activity of Sutton Harbour and the Barbican. This is a critical 'arm' of the city, hinged at either end by points of arrival by rail and by water. In the long term, the eventual removal of the rather ill-considered Staples building would create a broad sloping square of civic scale, providing an appropriate setting and approach for both Charles Church and the Barbican.

This is one of the key arcs of connection that are basic elements of the plan, making the link from the station and the University cultural quarter, through the new Drake's Circus development and continuing south down through Bretonside to Sutton Harbour and the Barbican.

The University

On the north-eastern boundary of the City Centre lies the University of Plymouth, where, once again, we discover the legacy of Abercrombie's plan has left a problematic relationship between two fundamental parts of the city. The combination of the scale and form of the highway arrangement, and the relegation of the pedestrian to subways wastes much of the potential for the energy of the University activity to influence and animate the city. Moreover, it is not only the University that connects with the city at this point, but also the neighbourhoods of Mutley and beyond.

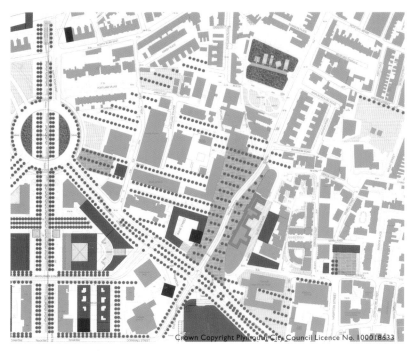

Crown Copyright Plymouth City Council Licence No. 100018633

52. **The University precinct**
Proposed public space on North Hill to unite the campus

Our proposal here illustrates two basic principles, which take forward ideas presented to us in the previous study by Llewelyn Davies,[8] and the work currently under way to produce a University Development Framework.[9]

Firstly, the connection between the two halves of the campus, at present bisected by the unnecessarily barriered highway of North Hill, should be improved. We firmly believe that the reduction of the width of North Hill and the removal of the central pedestrian barriers should be a priority for further detailed study. Existing strong façades on both sides of North Hill, coupled with the fine Sherwell Church and Portland Square building, provide the opportunity for a new public space focused on North Hill, providing a heart to the University and a catalyst to drive further interaction between the realms of public and institution. The proposed redevelopment of the Rowe Street site by the University is an important first stage of realising this vision, and must consciously contribute to its shaping.

Secondly, we must improve the connection of the University with the City Centre. The concept that is applied here is to rationalise the design of the current road, to present a human-scale street that will support pedestrian movement as well as vehicular. Our premise here is re-allocation of space through the creation of a boulevard with a central pedestrian walkway, which enables people to cross at points they choose, and stroll, run or rest in the central area. This is a road with a 30 mph speed limit, not a motorway, and two lanes of traffic travelling in one direction is safer to cross than two lanes of opposing traffic.

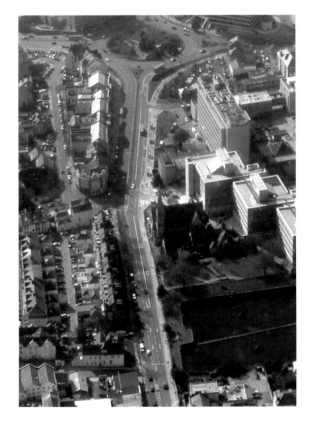

53. The University precinct
Existing open space provides an excellent basis for a high-quality environment

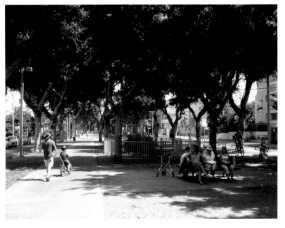

54. Rothschild Boulevard, Tel Aviv
A pedestrian highway that carries green space and people through the heart of the city

If the City Centre is to succeed as a destination for more than just shopping but also as a place to live, work, and play, then the perception and physical reality of the 'retail island' must be eroded. Nurturing diversity of uses, and breaking down the barriers to movement are key to ensuring that transformation can occur.

The capacity for change

At first glance, it may appear radical that our plan proposes the redevelopment of one-quarter of the City Centre area. Actually, the plan really places another layer – a spatial strategy – on top of areas already allocated for transformation in draft planning documents, and other sites identified by our team as suitable for redevelopment within the 20-year period allowed for the realisation of the vision. These are all sites that are capable of redevelopment at higher densities, in forms more appropriate to the needs of the city. The vision reflects upon this analysis and provides a strategic approach to appropriate blocks of development across the City Centre and adjacent areas. The development envelope has been assessed in relation to these footprint areas and approximation of building heights and suitable proportion of uses. It is important to note that the capacities have not been based upon ownership information; we have assumed that site assembly would be undertaken to fit the urban design principles outlined in the vision.

The City Centre benefits from a series of development initiatives that are in progress (Drake's Circus and Bretonside), developments that are nearing completion (the Travelodge at Derry's Cross, and student housing on Royal Parade and at Cobourg Street), and sites that have been assembled with emerging development proposals (Colin Campbell Court and the Civic Centre car-park). Our concern in looking at the implementation is to raise expectations for the City Centre as these welcome investments come forward. The vision makes clear that the key move for the regeneration of Plymouth is to reinvigorate the City Centre: this is the single most important element in transforming the image of the place.

In our analysis we have found strong division of function with the management of the City Centre. We feel that this has hampered an integrated process of regenerating the core. Division of function between highways, planning and urban design departments, landlords, bus operator, licensing authority and car-park operator has encouraged independent territories to act in competition with each other. There is a danger that a continuation of this approach could leave the City Centre forever languishing in the mire of the mediocre, and therefore our vision has posed a new and altogether braver future, one that befits the heritage of this proud waterside city.

New methodologies of partnership structures now exist within the regeneration industry, that align private sector and public sector interests, that respect the views of the community, that provide the critical new infrastructure of both transport and public space, that generate new possibilities of development use and form and that set new standards of design excellence. We return to these challenges in the final chapter and focus on possible options to investigate these integrated development vehicles further.

Armada Way

> The plan has two predominant axes – the one north and south being dominated by the Hoe on the south and by a large traffic circus in Cobourg Street in the north, which will form the main approach to the station and a focal point for city traffic. Thus, anyone entering the city from the railway or from the main bus station will get a magnificent impression of the expanse of business and civic centres and, at the same time, the Hoe beyond.[10]

Thus Abercrombie's vision for the spine of the city, Armada Way, 45 m wide and 1400 m long, which runs from the railway station to the Hoe. Both ends are about 30 m above sea level, and the route dips down to cross Royal Parade at about 10 m above sea level. Abercrombie's vision was for it to be a mainly pedestrian space, but incorporating traffic lanes running north-south.

The realisation of the proposal is somewhat disappointing: the complex topography raises North Cross roundabout as the perceived termination of the axis, leaving the station lost in the distance, marked only by an off-centre office building. Furthermore, as the route passes through the shopping centre, the legacy of various local interventions, coupled with the introduction of low-level vegetation, has obscured the very generous scale and identity of this majestic sweep through the townscape.

As a structuring element of the city, Armada Way is responsible for the connection and movement from the station to the waterfront, and indeed beyond the station to the north into Central Park.

Firstly, our proposal defines a new form for the station: a tall structure, glazed to the north and south, would provide a marker for the transport interchange and an invitation to explore the rolling townscape beyond. Access to the platforms would be provided from above, along with public access to the park area to the north. The forecourt area of the station retains the level of North Road, and is provided with a suitably urban feel by the introduction of a tall building on the east side, framing both station approach and the views of the station itself. Provision is also made for space to accommodate a coach and bus interchange, allowing seamless transfer to onward journeys.

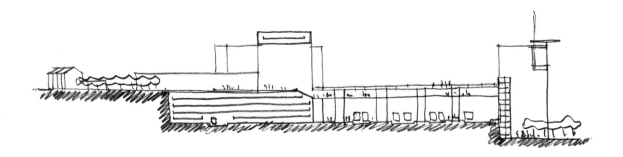

55. The railway station
Sketch section of proposal to lift the station to the level of city

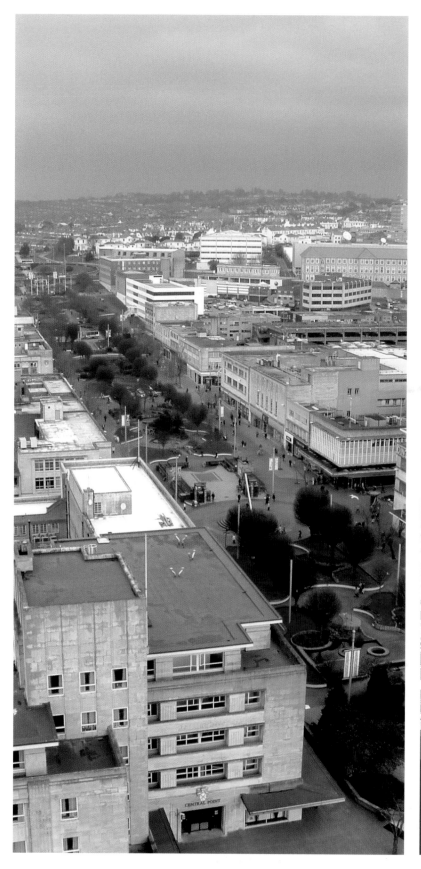
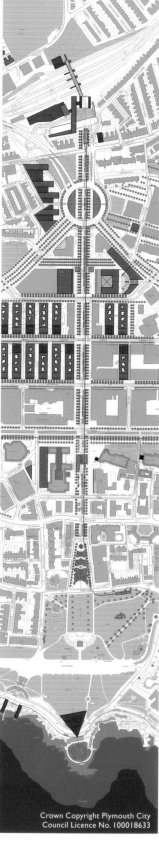

56, 57. Armada Way
The existing environment is cluttered, so that the significance of the link between the railway station and the
Hoe is lost. The proposed changes re-establish the importance of the spine

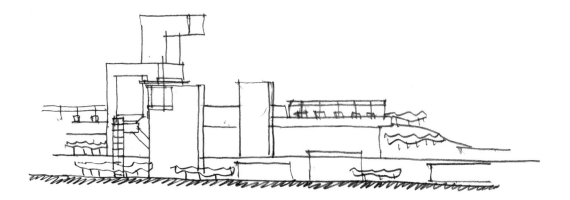

58. The railway station
The proposed station complex viewed from Central Park

North Cross roundabout is a difficult knot to untie in traffic terms, yet most agree that it is a poor use of land and a terrible pedestrian experience and gateway to the city. In principle, the approach is to engage and encroach upon the fragmented space here, rather than retreating with defensive anti-urban forms. Our plan proposes that Armada Way must continue, at grade, across the roundabout for both pedestrians and possible public transport. Car parking may be possible underneath this 'deck', although accessing it may prove difficult. Water features have been suggested on the east and west sides of the roundabout, for the purpose of part-shielding those in the centre from the noise and view of the surrounding traffic. To the west of North Cross, we have indicated a new building form as a long-term vision for densification in response to the development of the transport hub. This form is envisaged as employment-based and of an appropriate scale to respond to, and address, the context.

The sheer length and strategic function of Armada Way raises the question of how to improved the system of movement along its course. We feel it is important to retain the route as predominantly pedestrian, and propose that a new cohesive landscape strategy be developed, with an emphasis on clarity and flow, as opposed to the current obstructions. Regular lines of trees should be introduced to mark the formality and scale of the axis, and street furniture should be introduced as required to define and animate individual areas. We propose that the central area be kept clear of all obstructions, to allow for events, processions, markets etc., and advocate the preservation of a 6 m-wide lane on the eastern side for a future transport system. Where more carefully considered existing landscaping is found (e.g. between Royal Parade and Notte Street), it must be essentially retained within any new proposals.

A proposal exists for a new food pavilion to be located in Armada Way at the junction of New George Street and Cornwall Street, with a competition-winning design by a respected architecture practice. Whilst our strategy for the City Centre is based on diversification of the range of services available, we do not support the principle of disturbing this principal axis in a fragmentary way. The demand to provide this accommodation should be refocused into the process of redeveloping the adjacent city blocks.

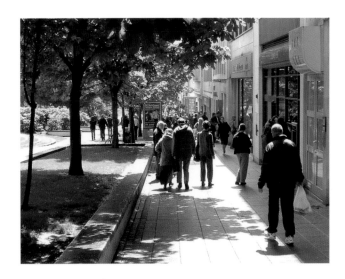

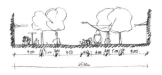

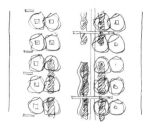

59, 60. Armada Way
The existing design crowds pedestrians at the edges. The proposed changes will improve the system of movement and civic scale

Where Armada Way meets Royal Parade we again encounter the legacy of obsolete thinking, with pedestrians channelled below one of the finest streets in Plymouth. Providing a generous surface-level crossing at this point should be a priority for the city, and would be a symbolic first expression of a new attitude to the relationship of pedestrians and vehicles in the City Centre.

We suggest that – as originally envisaged by Abercrombie – a water feature be installed to take advantage of the rising gradient of the Hoe. This will entice pedestrians to the water beyond, and also balance the water feature at North Cross.

At the termination of this axis we find the Dome, tucked away shyly over the lip of the Hoe. Our proposal here is to extend the influence of this rather lost building with a gallery extension that must both mark the termination of the axis, and retain views out to the water from the Hoe.

Sutton Harbour

Sutton Harbour lies to the west of the River Plym and east of the early settlement that hid unseen from the sea behind the headland known as the Hoe. There is a narrow strip of volcanic rock that created a natural breakwater which helped form Sutton Pool. The pier and present locks are located along the line of this natural breakwater. Brunel planned to put lock gates here in 1845, 150 years before they were finally built.[11] The geology of limestone, slate and volcanic rock, eroded over time, determined the geography of Sutton. The big tidal range of over 6 m allowed large ships to use this natural port.

These circumstances led to the foundation of the old city to the north-west of the Hoe headland. The flat lands to the east of the harbour between the Pool and the river Plym allowed the railway connections and hence industry and warehouses related to the port.

The Pool is Plymouth's fishing harbour, which is still commercially very active, with its new market on the east side providing fresh fish to many of the small restaurants around the harbour, as well as exports to the rest of the country. This authentic activity is the harbour's greatest charm, besides giving work to related workshops and warehouses. It is obvious that any development must be subsidiary to this historic and ongoing activity – it is the civilian equivalent of the naval bases in Devonport on the River Tamar to the west and along the Cattewater at the mouth of the River Plym to the east. Marine commerce remains active up the River Plym and helps sustain an important industrial and work area to the east of Sutton Harbour.

Beneath the shadow of the military Citadel, the old town neighbourhood of the Barbican retains the charm of its medieval past, having escaped damage during the war and the post-war development. Today it is Plymouth's main centre of attraction for citizens and tourists alike. The new lock has allowed an impressive marina to be installed in the Pool and there is now continuous demand for new accommodation around the harbour itself.

Sutton Harbour provides one of the key opportunities to carefully encourage economic vitality to spread outwards from the quaysides. There are three areas around Sutton Harbour that need careful architectural composition in order to avoid killing the attraction of the harbour edge – an edge threatened by the danger of creating a front wall of high buildings that block views to the harbour and prevent a perception that the areas behind also belong to it. These three areas – the East Quays, the link to the City Centre via the Charles Church memorial and Bretonside, and the wharves leading up to Fisher's Nose to the south – are the focus of our strategic approach and vision.

Although the Sutton Harbour Company has been, and still will be, the main economic driver, its property lines should not be the ultimate determining factor in the future street and building layout. The success of the Sutton Harbour model can inform the development of a sustainable surrounding neighbourhood.

Our approach has been informed by the early studies of the architects Form Design Group[12] and has developed in coordination with the Interim Planning Statements and Concept Plan prepared by the Sutton Partnership for the Local Development Framework.[13]

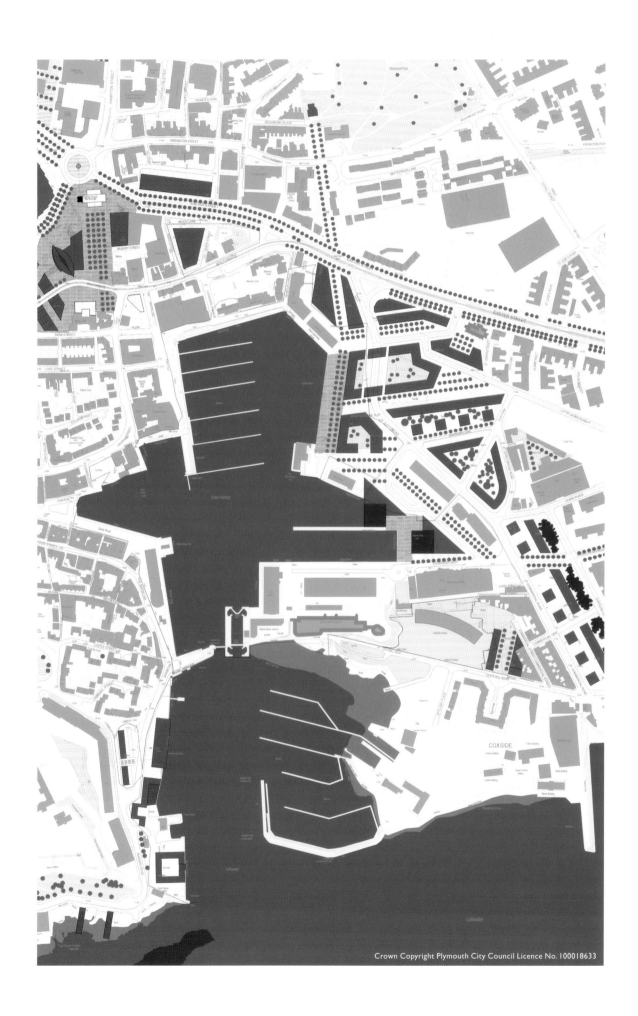

The East Quays

Keeping to the principle that the street reflects and reinforces the values of our society, then it is this public space and its form, contained between the edges of buildings, that must be considered first when examining the existing urban structure and its repair and extension in the area to the east of Sutton Harbour.

In order to consider this site as a whole, we must assume that some kind of land assembly has to be undertaken, either by direct acquisition of all the land by the public authority or by a series of agreements between the various landowners that allows a system of compensation between them. In the case of the East Quays we have respected in principle all existing constructions, with the exception of some industrial or warehouse sheds and at least one project known to have reached the stage of a formal planning application.

The proposals follow the main spine routes identified by the Local Development Framework (LDF). Sutton Road runs roughly southwards from the main Exeter road (A 374) by the fish market, then after crossing the Barbican approach road from the east leads on to the Cattedown industrial area that faces the bend of Cattewater. To the north-south Sutton Road we must add the east-west Barbican approach road, which follows the former tracks of an old railway line through a cutting and ends at the fish market and aquarium, finally allowing pedestrians to cross over the new lock gates to the Barbican on the west side. These two streets form the main street structure of the East Quays and their crossing is where the new centre should be generated.

It is near this crossing and facing the Pool on the Coxside inlet that we propose to situate two high-rise buildings of 18 floors, with an extended triangular ground-floor base that follows an access street parallel to Sutton Road. These towers will give a metropolitan scale to the east side of Sutton Harbour and form a visual landmark from the Barbican approach. Together with the nearby fish market and Aquarium, these two towers, containing offices, dwellings, hotel, etc., will be sufficient to establish an active meeting place by the quays.

Our main objective is to give the East Quays not only a neighbourhood identity but a metropolitan one so that on the one hand, people from all over the city will be attracted to go there, while on the other hand, the possibility of a landmark building in the splendid waterside setting could attract a European consortium to establish its head offices here.

Sutton Road, which runs parallel to the Quays, should be the spine connecting a series of side streets that will allow the clear connection of the whole area with the harbour to be perceived. This follows the traditional pattern of streets giving access to the waterside that is found in most active inner harbours or towns that lie on navigable rivers. It is suggested that the advantages of this system would not only enhance the living conditions of those living behind the waterfront, but also substantially increase the inherent property values.

61. **Sutton Harbour**
The proposed plan

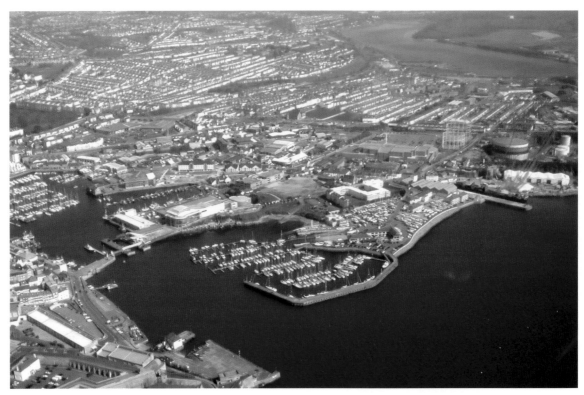

62. **Sutton Harbour**
Where a vibrant mix of living, working, and leisure has already been achieved

The side street that leads from the end of the North Quay to St John's church, should be a broad street (30 m wide) with a wide pavement to the north side to capture the sun in a sheltered place (like some of the old streets in Philadelphia). This street could attract local shops, banks, etc., to form a strongly identified social space for the residents of the neighbourhood, away from the tourist edge of the quays. This axis from the Pool to the church would be clearly visible from the West Quays.

Other parallel side streets could contain a varied morphology, including a large courtyard building with bridge buildings over Sutton Road to create a private community garden. The rest of the side streets have been adapted to the existing industrial streets.

The quays themselves also need attention. The Marrowbone Slip, for example, could be filled in to create continuity along the quays. The quays themselves should be at least 30 m deep, similar to the successful West Quays, to provide space for sheltering trees and shrubs. This would allow restaurants and bars to put tables and chairs outdoors in the summer and erect provisional glazed rooms in winter. With careful design, the quays could also absorb a certain amount of temporary car parking. The heights of the buildings should not be more than six floors, with perhaps a recessed penthouse.

In front of the Barbican Leisure Park with its cinemas and bowling alley, and between Gashouse Lane adjoining the service entrances, and Commercial Road, a continuation of Sutton Road, one of the side streets, a line of row houses with smaller pavilion-type housing could make this an attractive high density, low rise area, with both public parks and private terraces.

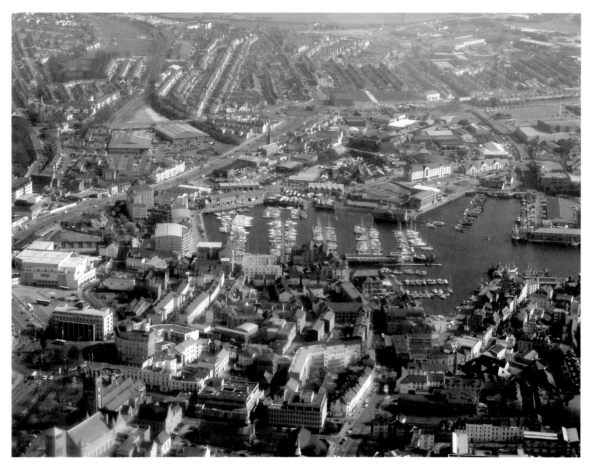

63. **Sutton Harbour**
The opportunity to spread the benefit of the waterside eastwards into adjacent communities

There are two important elements of the infrastructure that must be carefully studied and valued for their social importance. The first is a pedestrian connection between the hillside communities surrounding Beaumont Park and the waterfront. This would provide a pleasant tree-lined walk to the quay of Marrowbone Slip and on to the China House tavern on the waterfront. This is not an incidental urban design suggestion; it is a fundamental feature that forms an integral part of sewing the city together. The proposed development at this area must be adjusted to allow this pedestrian connection.

The second concerns the nearby East End, on the eastern side of Cattedown Road, which is being intelligently renovated and restored. This can be linked to Sutton Harbour by extending St John's Road in the East Quays area to bridge over the sunken Gdynia Way and connect with Maidstone Avenue in the East End. The bridge would have to rise gently over Gdynia Way to make this possible.

If development in the East Quays is to be successfully integrated into the extended centre of Plymouth, these two links with the neighbouring districts are essential. The cost of these public works should be partly paid for out of the increased land values of the East Quays area of Sutton Harbour. The total built area could be in the region of 150,000 sq m, or the equivalent of 1,500 dwellings, depending on the amount of employment space provided.

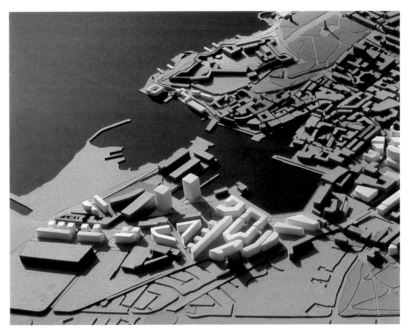

64. Sutton Harbour
Model of proposals, illustrating links to Sutton Harbour from the Barbican Approach, Exeter Street and Beaumont Park

Link to the City Centre

The link to the City Centre is focused on two adjoining areas: the Bretonside bus station and Charles Church, both of which are discussed in the City Centre chapter of this report.

Critically, it is recommended that the future development should provide several pedestrian routes between Exeter Street and Bretonside, to create the perception of a large public square containing several buildings at least six floors high related to Essex Street. It would be appreciated if an additional visual link could be established between Buckwell Street and the spire of Charles Church. These visual links will be completed by widening Tin Lane to align with How Street.

Charles Church has already been referred to, but the importance of the restoration of its setting and impact must be underlined. It should function not only as a memorial but also as an essential knuckle in the proposed articulated link between the Barbican/Sutton Harbour and the City Centre. This implies the difficult task of recovering the recently-built Staples and Bingo building. Sometimes the removal of one building can do more for the well-being of the city than the erection of 50 new ones. This is a challenging aspiration that will require a step-change in market conditions to drive the transformation, or the long-term redundancy of the structure. Observing how the will of other cities and their citizens have achieved similar objectives elsewhere, gives us hope that within the timespan of this vision this objective will be achieved. The new, sloping public square, lined with trees, would provide an ideal place for a sheltered open market, an activity attractive to both the Barbican/Sutton Harbour and the City Centre itself.

A little bit of surgery will be needed to widen Tin Lane which links How Street with the North Quay, but this would be well worth while. This has been pointed out to us by local residents, and we welcome the suggestion.

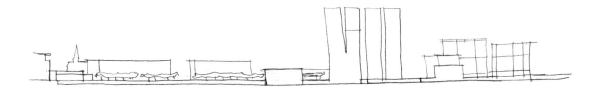

65. Sutton Harbour
Suggested profile of the East Quay, avoiding a barrier to the communities beyond

Fisher's Nose

This proposal is inspired by the way in which previous buildings huddled around the slipways and wharves, right up against the water.

On Commercial Wharf, we could create a ramped entrance from the north. The wharf could accommodate the proposed marine investigation laboratories, housing different institutions, with exhibition areas for the visiting public. There would still be sufficient space for the ferry services.

Behind the Commercial Wharf, between Lambhay Hill and Madeira Road, the existing car-park should be replaced by terraced housing stepping down the hillside with residential car parking underneath. Around the slipway a building configuration similar to the former constructions could house a hotel.

On the car-park at Fisher's Nose a square block, with a court open to the water with steps, built to the scale of Plymouth's military constructions, could contribute to a fine architectural monument to the entrance to Sutton Harbour. It is envisaged that it would house private dwellings.

On-street car parking could be increased along Madeira Road beyond Fisher's Nose, with a slight widening to allow car parking perpendicular to the traffic flow (which would have to be a one-way circulation westwards).

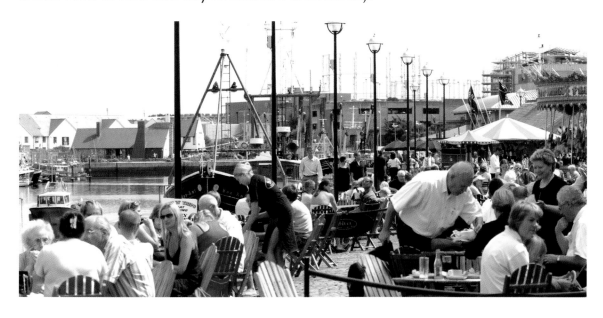

66. Sutton Harbour
A lively and vibrant urban waterfront

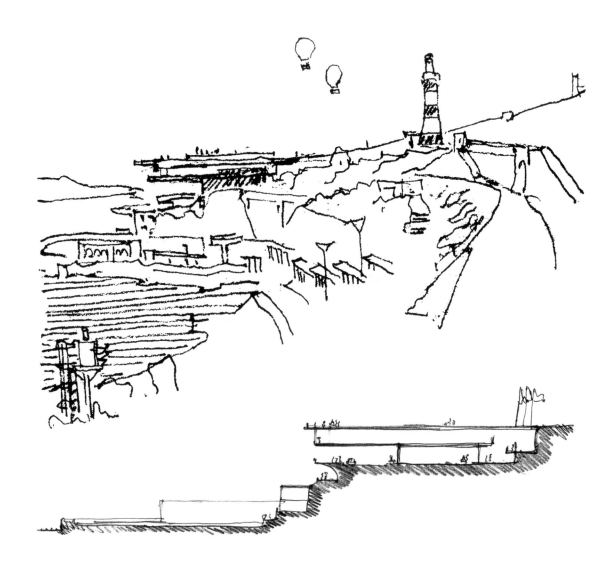

67, 68. The Waterfront
Proposed new gallery above the Dome, show in perspective (top) and section

The Waterfront

We have already explored the strategic importance of Plymouth's key waterfront development sites, Millbay and Sutton Harbour, and the critical issue of how their development might influence regeneration of areas further inland, particularly through improved physical connection with the City Centre. However, the relationship between Plymouth and the waterfront stretches far beyond these two amphitheatres of activity – although the buzz they generate does serve to draw attention to the deadness of the spaces in between. We envisage the Hoe fulfilling a new pivotal role on the waterfront, as both a connecting element and an attractive destination in its own right.

Our plan therefore offers four concepts or considerations for the Hoe foreshore, which will strengthen this coastal edge and improve the image of the existing route along Madeira Road and Hoe Road. These proposals aim to stimulate movement, drawing people along this unrivalled coastline, and secure moments of rest, protection and interest along the route.

Access

The Hoe, through its very nature as a prominent geographical feature, presents access difficulties to both vehicles and pedestrians. Our observations confirm that, despite its central location within the wider city, the Hoe foreshore receives many of its visitors by private vehicle. It is an amenity popular with many of the older citizens of Plymouth, so parking provision is vital, yet the current arrangement of the area does not encourage those who can walk to do so.

The first consideration therefore would be to study the section of the road, to investigate the possibility of providing more car parking facing the sea. This would allow more people to have access to the Hoe and also allow viewing of the Sound and its theatre of shipping from the car on wet and windy days.

A new focus

The second consideration is to establish two major attractions – one cultural, the other scientific – that will draw greater movement to the area. The Dome, which holds such a commanding position in the landscape, has had only moderate commercial success, we propose a remodelling that would extend it, adding a 1,500 sq m triangular gallery above for temporary exhibitions. Perhaps this could be dedicated to the painter Sir Joshua Reynolds, a Plymouth citizen who became the first president of the Royal Academy. It might form a catalyst for co-operation and exchange between the RA and a new institution in Plymouth. Secondly, the topography of the western edge of the Hoe provides a hollow at West Park, which could accommodate a striking pavilion, set within the landscape and enjoying a stunning aspect across the water. Abercrombie considered a similar use for this site in his plan for Plymouth; it is time now to restate this bold proposition, and show that the cityscape at the waterfront is defined by more than just the Holiday Inn and other tall buildings.

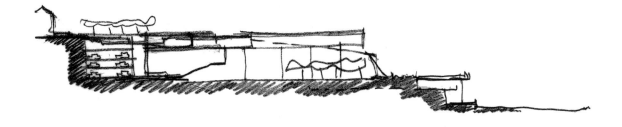

69. The Waterfront
Section through the proposed pavilion in the hollow of West Park

70, 71, 72 (Overleaf). **Proposals for the Waterfront**

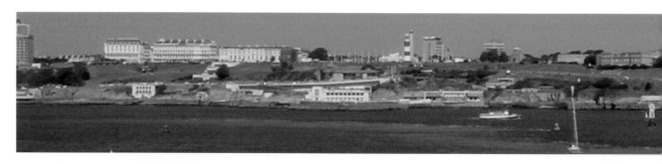

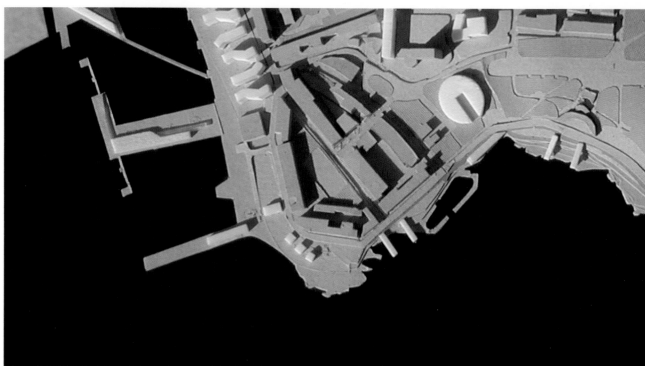

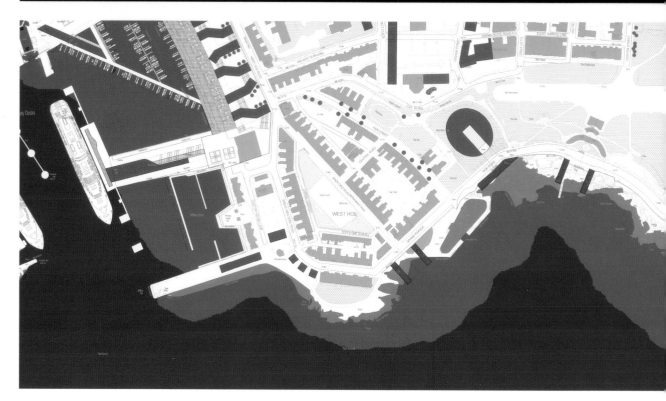

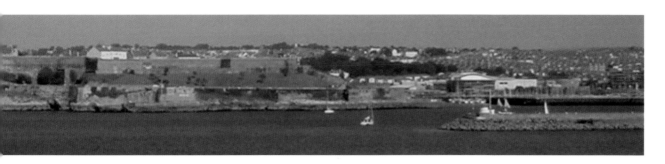

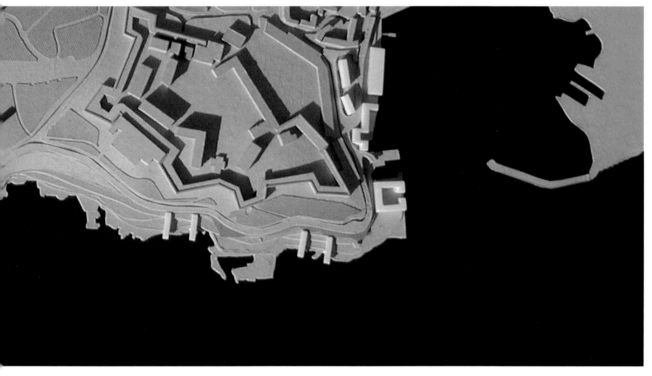

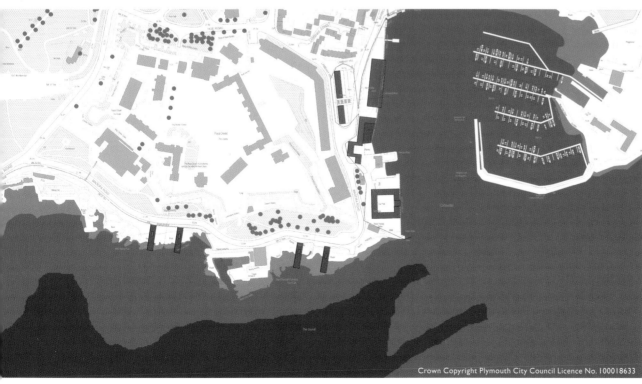

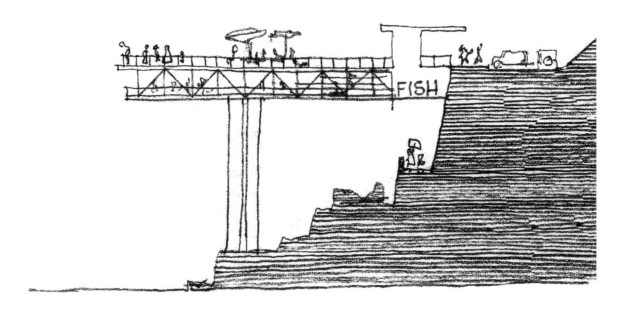

73. **The Waterfront**
Proposed piers projecting into the water

A new façade for the city

The third consideration is to improve the image and definition of the Hoe in the evening and at night. At present, its isolation from the pulse of the city at night gives the area an unsafe and unwelcoming feeling inconsistent with its beauty and potential. We would like to see a lighting scheme for the length of the Hoe foreshore that would make it visible from the surrounding hillsides and mark this historic place as an evening and events destination for all. It may be possible, for example, to redesign the footpath and extend it so that its surface would light up as one walked along it, or on other occasions be lit up completely to form a ribbon of light. The natural curves of the coastline would ensure that the lighting could be seen from all directions.

The fourth consideration would be to construct projecting piers with their decks at road level and with restaurants or cafés hung underneath, providing splendid views over the Sound. There could be a mix of popular fast food outlets with more sophisticated restaurants, offering the variety required to make this a place for all. A wealth of historic structures is embedded in the coastline; these must, like Tinside Lido, be given a chance to flourish once more. But needs and aspirations have moved on since these elements were constructed, and we therefore raise the question: how might a contemporary intervention along this stretch look?

74 (facing page, top). **The Waterfront**
Suggested network of water transport

75 (facing page, bottom). **Plymouth**
Proposed urban structure integrating the centre with the waterfront and adjacent neighbourhoods

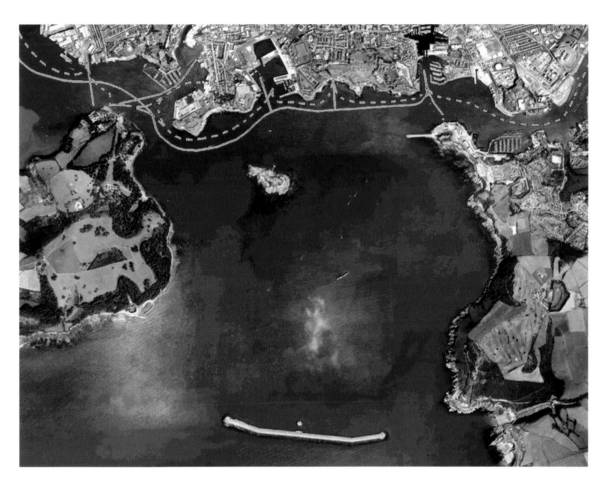

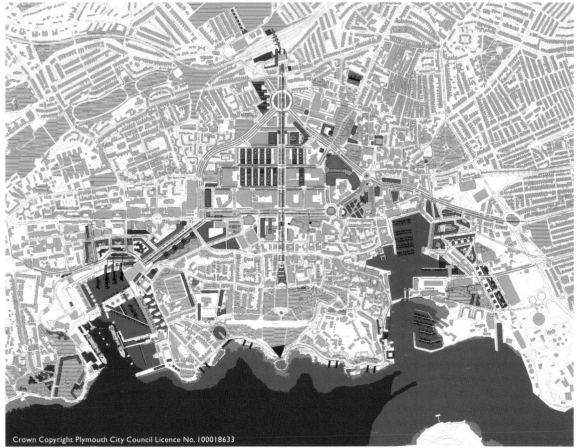

Notes

1. Lacey Hickie Caley Architects, Millbay Regeneration Strategy, 2003.

2. Cullen, op. cit., p. 114.

3. SWERDA is the agency responsible for promoting the economic success of the region.

4. English Partnerships is the national regeneration agency, helping the Government to achieve sustainable growth in England.

5. Watson and Abercrombie, op. cit., p. 71.

6. English Heritage Urban Panel Review Paper, March 2002.

7. Plymouth City Council, Plymouth City Centre Precinct Urban Design Framework, 2001.

8. Llewelyn Davies, University of Plymouth Draft Development Framework, 2002.

9. Plymouth University Partnership, *Goals for the Future of the University of Plymouth*, Consultation Draft, July 2003.

10. Watson and Abercrombie, op. cit., p. 70.

11. Gill, C., *Sutton Harbour*, Devon Books, 1997.

12. Form Design Group, Development at Harbour Avenue, 2003.

13. Plymouth City Council, Sutton Harbour East Interim Planning Statement, 2003.

Chapter Five
Recommendations

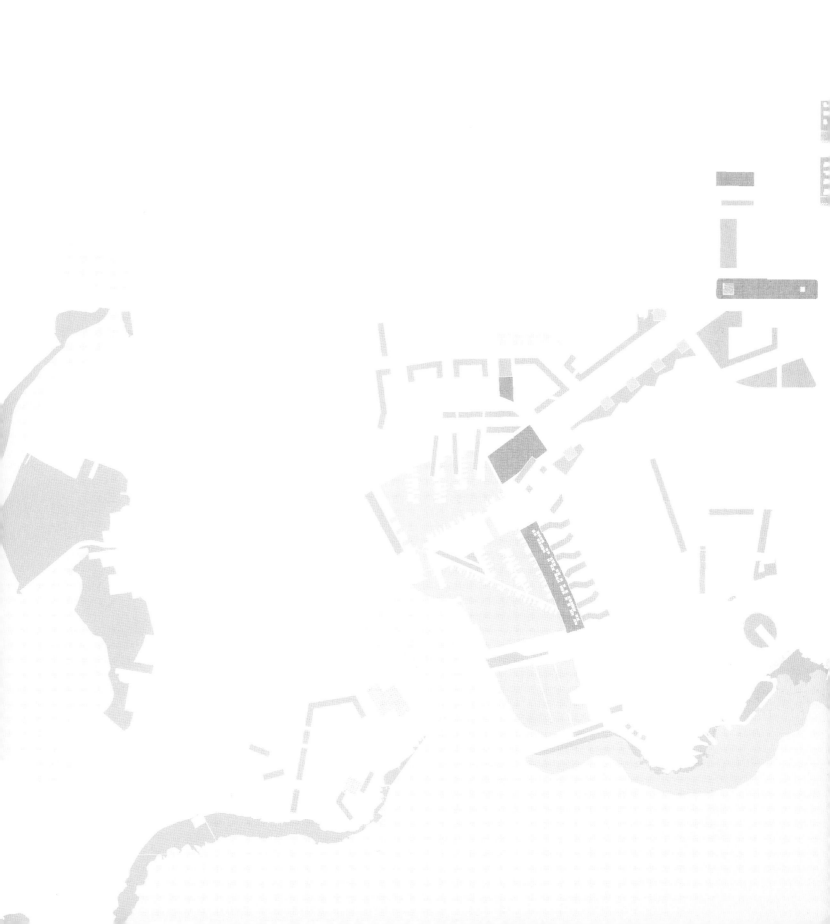

City-wide vision – connecting the opportunities

The plans presented here outline our vision for the regeneration of the city of Plymouth. It is a vision that sets out a future for the city that is built upon its waterfront setting, its heritage and its capacity for consolidation and expansion. Plymouth, one of the largest urban areas in the South West, has significant capacity for regeneration and intensification in the areas and neighbourhoods that have been described in our work. A fundamental principle in the implementation of our vision is to provide mechanisms that connect the areas of opportunity to each other and across the city.

It therefore follows that the implementation strategy required must harness the existing private sector development activity in the city and facilitate partnership arrangements with public sector agencies that will ensure that these connections are made for the benefit of the entire city. This is a flexible and deliverable approach that uses the physical vision as a base to demonstrate an overall future structure for the city. It builds upon private and public project partnerships to facilitate each part of these strategies. Within the central area of Plymouth the vision has accommodated existing development initiatives and has sought to ensure in the delivery process that they are aligned with its principles. This approach provides 'early win' opportunities for the vision, giving credibility and confidence to the wider community. Later stages will require wider community and public sector funding support.

Population and economic growth

One of the key tenets of the vision is intensification. We have quoted the existing population statistics for both the urban and the travel-to-work catchment area, and have suggested that over the next 20 years it is reasonable to expect that the city could develop to an urban population of between 300,000 and 350,000. The plan explains how this intensification can be shaped by physical developments on the ground. The vision is built upon sites that support the wider urban design aspiration. They have all been identified for potential future development in local plans and by local stakeholders. The total development footprint of the plan is approximately 950,000 sq m of new floor space, allocated to a mix of uses, from which we could expect to achieve between 8,000 and 8,500 residential units.

Statistics from the National Land Use Database (2003)[1] confirm that Plymouth has 129 hectares of previously developed vacant land and buildings, and 26 hectares of derelict land and buildings which support the capacity being suggested in the vision. Indeed, this is the highest 'brownfield' capacity in the region, and further capacity for development will come from the opportunities of redevelopment of the existing stock. The new uses generated for the defence accommodation as it becomes redundant will also provide redevelopment opportunities.

In describing the vision we have identified opportunities for densification in the City Centre by changes in the form of the buildings sitting within the Abercrombie urban grid. The regeneration of redundant port and naval areas has and will create further development opportunities, including Sutton Harbour, Royal William Yard, Devonport, and Millbay, with more to come over time. The vision has shown how the connector pieces of the city joining the current disparate areas will also become opportunities for development.

In reviewing the economy it is clear that Plymouth is a sub-regional shopping centre and plays a major role as an employment centre for the region, with 70% of jobs in the city being in the service sector. It also has a major university located in the north of the City Centre, with a 20,000 student population.

We believe that the key to the development of the economy is for the city to increase its attractiveness as a place for work, living and play. This vision explains how Plymouth, with its extraordinary setting, should attract businesses and residents migrating to the South West in search of a better quality of life. However, most of the household growth need for Plymouth is generated from within the existing population and therefore the vision needs to also respond the needs of those living in Plymouth now, to stem the flow of outward migration of the younger age groups. The improvement and regeneration of the City Centre has to be the magnet for this movement, and growth of population will assist in the positioning of Plymouth in the wider context of the regional city within Europe.

Competing urban centres within the United Kingdom and Europe are severely constrained by their historic environment, limited building stock and constrained surrounding landscape, which all limit their potential for growth. Despite current government policy on Growth Areas and the impact of the Barker Report[2] we believe that further New Town development on greenfield sites is still considered unsustainable in both public opinion and government policy, and will only be permitted as a last resort. The reworking of the Plymouth urban area and the opportunities for its expansion on brownfield land therefore offer a distinct advantage to the city.

This land opportunity, the waterside setting and the vision represent the springboard for the economic and physical regeneration of the city.

City management – responsibilities, strengths and weaknesses

In considering an implementation strategy for the city vision we have looked at the various management structures already in place and examined their ability to lead and deliver the vision. Currently the city operates through the local private and public institutions and their managements. These include Plymouth City Council, the SWERDA, EP, the Sutton Harbour Company, the University of Plymouth, and the Ministry of Defence. Rather usefully, these are also the institutions that control the key landholdings in the City: the City Centre estate is in the hands of the City Council, Millbay is owned by the SWERDA and EP, and the North Hill area belongs to the University. When considering the implementation strategy for the plan, it is reassuring to note that these key public and private sector partners are in a position to unlock the land base that is critical to the vision.

However, we have become aware during the course of our study that there are historic divisions between different elements within the city. The implementation strategy will need to address this issue and find processes and structures that join these disparate parts together to make possible the wider transformation of the city. During the period of this study, Plymouth 2020 Partnership has provided just such community-wide involvement. If the vision is to be successfully implemented, a similar body will need to lead the project forward in an open way that builds on the support and good faith of this city-wide community.

In all projects that look to the future, initiatives that are already under way need to be accommodated within proposals. Indeed, the vision we have outlined has been informed by the development initiatives that are under way. Thus the first stages of the implementation will include the Rowe Street development by the University, and the Drake's Circus redevelopment by P&O Developments. Despite arriving on the scene late in the negotiations over these developments, we have been able to influence both of these initiatives. The University's commitment to quality led them to welcome our input, and we were able to assist in both the preparation of the urban design brief for the campus and the selection of architects to the Rowe Street project. In relation to the Drake's Circus development, we support the investment in City Centre shopping that reinforces the economic heart of the city, and provides for 24-hour permeability from north to south across and through the Abercrombie grid.

In our opinion, both of these developments on the eastern axis of the City Centre will assist the realisation of the proposed redevelopment of the block between Mayflower Street and Cornwall Street as the 'Drake's Circus effect' fans out across the City Centre. Other imminent investments in the city have the opportunity to follow such commitment; the developments of Bretonside, Colin Campbell Court and the Derry's Cross area are at various stages, but they all can and should reflect the key principles of permeability and design that lie at the root of the vision.

Critical to the delivery of the vision will be the development of Millbay. The report and the plans prepared by MBM focus proposals that have been the subject of initial discussion with key parties. This development needs to maintain a relationship with the entire vision, and its implementation must take into account the infrastructure connections along Bath Street, the redevelopment of the Pavilions and the construction of Battery Street, which will provide alternative access to the port traffic. The possibility of cross-funding between residential development and the commercial elements of the scheme has been outlined in Chapter Four. The proposed Sutton Harbour development extends the successful regeneration to the east of the harbour, and is a partnership of interests between the Sutton Harbour Company and Plymouth City Council.

In our opinion the key element that will assist the implementation of the plan is the reinforcement of the waterfront. Whilst other cities and towns in the South West enjoy their beaches, Plymouth is a waterfront city in the tradition of Liverpool, Glasgow or Genoa. In the regeneration of these comparable cities the process of change has focused on the recovery of the waterfront and has usually involved the remaking of port areas and the opening-up of access. In Plymouth the proposal is to open up the waterfront by the development of Millbay to the west and the Barbican to the east, using the Hoe as the connector between the two. The improvement of Armada Way will link the Hoe through to the City Centre. There will, however, remain a need to support the development of port activity and other marine commercial activity, whilst seeking to realise the vision of opening up the waterfront for all the people of Plymouth.

Agencies, institutions and leadership

In the process of the study we have led a series of stakeholder seminar sessions, which have identified some of the key players in the City. In addition to these sessions we have conducted meetings with individual participants. These have included groups representing the City Centre Partnership, Associated British Ports, Sutton Harbour, the University of Plymouth, and the P & O developments. We have met in a separate session groups of local architects and their local developers and investors to understand the finer grain aspects of development in the city, the residential schemes, the student housing schemes and other aspects of new development initiatives. In further sessions we have met representatives of Plymouth City Council, the Regional Development Agency (SWERDA) and Government Office for the South West (GOSW). In addition we have met key representatives of the resident community, the business community and the arts community. With the study's support team, consisting of staff from Plymouth 2020 and Plymouth City Council, we have discussed forward plan policies which have included planning, highways, transport and urban design, special policy and emerging policy guidance. We made interim presentations of our plan early in the summer to keep the wider community informed of our approach.

In this series of information gathering, initial debate and analysis sessions we have learnt that Plymouth has an active development market for urban residential development, predominantly on waterside sites or sites with views of the water. This includes the recently completed Royal William Yard, new developments at Sutton Harbour, and new residential schemes around the Hoe. The city also has an active market for retail, expressed in the Drake's Circus retail development by P&O, and for mixed use, expressed through the Bretonside development by Henry Boot.

Further development activity in the City Centre includes new buildings for the University of Plymouth, a recently completed new hotel, new student housing, and developments at Colin Campbell Court and the Ballard Centre. In all of these projects we have observed an active development process at work, in which design and development briefs generated by Plymouth City Council from its Urban Design Framework have been used to guide and ensure high-quality development on these sites.

The formation of the City Centre Partnership has paved the way for the City Centre to be included as a 'business improvement district' pathfinder project. This local leadership and initiative is exemplary.

We have seen leadership of local projects well established. The University is generating high-quality architecture and urban design proposals reflecting its high aspirations for their campus and the creation of the cultural quarter alongside. The recently completed science and teaching facility by Fielden, Clegg and Bradley is of very high quality, and the current architectural competition for the Rowe Street arts facility continues this investment in architecture. This leadership is also exemplary.

The development of Sutton Harbour by the Sutton Harbour Company, working in partnership with Plymouth City Council, has demonstrated a long-term commitment to a regeneration process emerging from the transformation of the old harbour and its fishing fleet. The creation of marinas, the half-tide basin, the Aquarium and the waterside apartments, restaurants and bars, along with the associated enhancement of the public realm and sense of place, is a major success story for the city. We have taken it as a starting-point for our vision of city-wide regeneration. Adding and developing linkage from this successful quarter of the city back to the City Centre and along the waterfront to Millbay are key elements of our vision.

The vision has been prepared on the intelligence and knowledge of these existing development projects, which have formed a foundation to the plan and a starting point for its range and scope, taking the city onward through the next 20 years. The individual project leadership that has driven these exemplary and pioneering projects forward needs to be replicated at the centre of this vision, to provide and maintain the momentum that will drive through these individual projects within the city-wide perspective. Whilst to date individual leaders have focused on specific projects, and benefited from good relations with the City Council to support these initiatives, the vision needs the step change in thinking and leadership that will take up the challenge of the regeneration and development of the entire City Centre and its relevant Strategic Opportunity Areas to realise the aspirations presented in this report.

We have described in this report the process by which the vision was developed and the 'reality check' that has been taken throughout the study period to ensure that the vision has grown organically out of the city of Plymouth and out of the reality of its development potential. In following that methodology we have produced a plan that is designed to meet current conditions and to provide links between pioneering developments in order that the great waterside city of Plymouth may aspire to taking its place among the principal regional centres of the UK and Europe.

The implementation of the vision needs leadership across the constituencies of the city. The approach must be one of partnership between all the different interests in the city that we have identified in this report. The work of the 2020 Partnership in promoting and supporting the study, in generating involvement from across all the elements of the city, and in acting as a local strategic partner, is a blueprint for the partnership approach that needs to be at the centre of any suitable delivery vehicle.

The partnership vehicle must fulfil a wider administrative role. It will need to secure commitment from public sector and private sector partners the partners to the realisation of the plan, and agreement between them to work together to deliver the plan. It needs to become a legal entity, one that can hold property, enter into contracts, and operate at arm's length to the local authority. The partners to this implementation vehicle need to agree to concede powers and responsibility and transfer land into the legal entity for it to begin its work.

Examples of such delivery vehicles are outlined below. There are three current formats: Urban Regeneration Companies (URCs), Millennium Communities (MCs) and Strategic Joint Venture (SJVs).

Urban Regeneration Companies

The URC, whilst not the only method of carrying forward the vision, is both a powerful and flexible tool that is tailored to local conditions and circumstances. The role of an URC is to realise the latent development and economic opportunities of an area in a comprehensive way and to raise investor confidence to the point where its physical regeneration becomes self-sustaining.

A consulting report to DTLR described the role of URCs as follows:

> URCs are a mechanism that is principally focused on one aspect of the problems facing an

area – its physical and associated economic regeneration URCs need to create a favourable climate into which the private sector will commit investment programmes for renewal.

The following criteria are used to evaluate this support:

- Full commitment and involvement by the key partners

- A close and effective working relationship with the local authority

- Getting the local strategy right and communicating it widely

- Appointing a highly effective Chair, Board, Chief Executive and Executive team. The Board should comprise key decision makers and influential individuals

- Developing a prioritised programme with clear implementation arrangements

- Effectively involving and engaging stakeholders

- Influencing the investment decisions of partners, other public sector organisations and importantly private sector investors

- Integrating with other initiatives and establishing a clear agreement on roles and responsibilities

- Establishing a positive momentum, through early high profile projects that are successfully delivered, and maintaining the momentum

- High quality standards in terms of design and architecture.

Millennium Communities

The second vehicle is the Millennium Communities, an initiative being led by EP. The recent announcement of the appointment of Urban Splash as lead developers for the New Islington project in East Manchester is an example of this programme, which started with the Millennium Villages at Greenwich and Allerton Bywater outside Leeds, and has announced a further Millennium Community at Hastings. The programme is administered by EP and is based upon quite defined pockets of 'brownfield' land which can be clearly defined as development opportunies, but ones in which the public sector needs to take a lead to promote the investment, with the private sector alongside. They are seen as opportunities to marry private sector entrepreneurial effort to public sector land holdings. These communities are a competitive allocation and EP would need to be consulted to discover whether Plymouth is eligible to be an approved MC.

Strategic Joint Venture

The third model is a Strategic Joint Venture initiative, whereby EP aim to bring their own skills and expertise together with those of local authorities and RDAs to focus on the local delivery of development strategies that provide 'sustainable urban regeneration' and makes 'the best use of surplus land and buildings'.

Other vehicles include Urban Development Corporations (UDCs), among other local partnership arrangements. Clearly, it is now essential that EP be consulted for their advice on suitable delivery vehicles for this project, as it fulfils the terms of their remit from the Office of the Deputy Prime Minister (ODPM), namely to '[unlock] the potential of public sector property'.

In addition to the advice of EP, this overall report should now be widely consulted upon, in particular with the key agencies operating within the city, to seek an agreement in principle to work in partnership to deliver this vision across the city. The will to work together in a spirit of co-operation with an agreement on leadership and on asset transfer to a new vehicle is the first and most important step towards the realisation of the plan. The final shape of the vehicle that delivers the plan will properly remain the subject of future investigation and debate. The purpose of this study has been to set an aspiration for the future shape of the city and to encourage commitment to and debate about on the part of all participants, public and private. The vision of the future we set before you is encouraging, challenging and deliverable.

The wider context of the 'vision' strategy

Throughout the developed world we observe the same conditions in the form and development of our mature cities: their economic stability changes, some develop apace, while others seem to wane. Economists over the past 30–40 years have examined this situation in some detail. They have explained that manufacturing has moved to economies that offer the greatest cost benefit to the manufacturer and permit him to take advantage of the best price to sell his goods on the global market. Any city with an economy based on a single, traditional, manufacturing industry will suddenly find itself without its major employer.

This has led to the development of wider, more diverse and more sustainable city economies, we talk today of the 'knowledge economy', the 'shopping economy', the 'tourist economy', the 'financial services economy' and the '24-hour economy'. All of these economic models tend to locate themselves within our urban centres, where they are grafted onto an existing infrastructure of buildings, roads and public spaces. They are the means of replacing and renewing the redundant fabric of the city.

New economies come into being through the various forces of regeneration. They start with the focus on redundant stock, driving the cost down, which in turn creates the opportunity for financial investment and entrepreneurial action. This is supported by public sector action, be it grant aiding, pump priming, tax breaks, new infrastructure or new forms of city management.

The fundamental point that sits behind the Plymouth vision is that it is the blueprint for the city to change. In this minute and simplified demonstration of the economic rationale we set the context of the city. We argue that this is a city that can, should and must change over the next decades. We have identified opportunities for the city to densify and expand its urban population and to attract the diversity of employer and economy that will support its economic growth.

The vision has been proposed as a response to the physical form of the city, to the existing policy frameworks of the city, and to the development opportunities that have been found. Much has been written in this report of the quality of the city, its unique and fortunate position with its extensive waterfront and its location between the popular and overcrowded areas of south Devon and south Cornwall. What this points to is the opportunity for this city to meet its potential by developing that attraction, transforming its image and making itself irresistible to the kind of fleet-footed, diverse

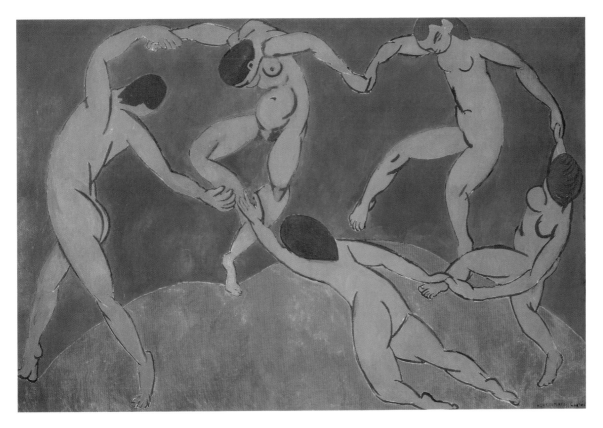

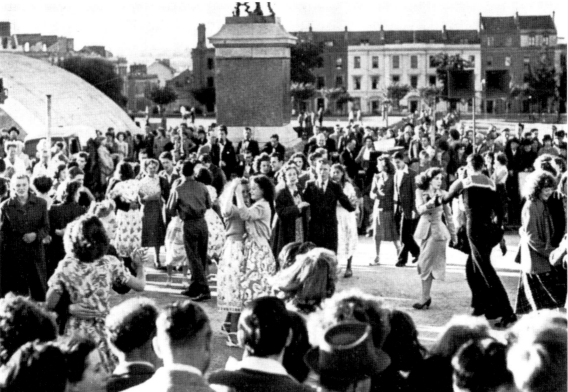

Have we the chance to dance again?

economic activity that could critically transform Plymouth and reposition it at the economic centre of the South West region.

The vision sets out the possibilities for the city, the ways of connecting its divided neighbourhoods, the blueprint to make the whole more than the sum of the parts. It is based upon the reality of what we have found, it is logical and realisable. However, it will not come about by itself. It needs political and business leadership, it needs to retain quality, it needs to stimulate the imagination and to surprise the local population. It needs a flowering of idea, of enterprise and of identity. It is a vital first step, it is robust, it represents a direction to be followed.

The city can take a voyage to the future, it can transform itself into a vibrant mixed-use culture, it can take advantage of its setting, it can expand and extend, it can take new buildings; they can be high, they can be low, they can be contemporary or contextual. They need in all places and at all times to be of high quality and beautiful. The plan must therefore be used with care. Do not allow it to stultify development or activity: it is a possibility, it is a wide picture of a future, it should and can permit huge variation in activity, encouraging individual responses that build into a coherent whole.

The city must have the confidence to sustain the vision, no matter what pressures are placed upon it as a result of any feeding frenzy among its developer friends. An intensified city means that parties have a renewed and different sense of responsibility towards each other and to their city. Each developer has a chance of making a heroic contribution to the city. Each development matters, each must build up to the connected, high-quality transformation that the vision articulates.

The political leadership is welcome, the administration participation is essential, the business community commitment is powerful, the agency partnerships impressive. The project now needs a champion – not to regulate or dictate, but to encourage, to release the local energy, to build momentum and convince the citizens of Plymouth to participate in their own future by embracing the vision we have laid before them.

Notes

1. www.nlud.org.uk.

2. Barker, K. *Delivering Stability. Securing our future housing needs*, London: HM Treasury, 2004.

Image Credits

Every effort has been made to trace the owners of illustrations. We would welcome contact from anyone who has not been mentioned so that they can be acknowledged in any future edition.

Ajuntamento de Barcelona: 13, 48; AZ Urban Studio: 25, 54; British Library: 8, 9; CPRE/Countryside Agency: 3; James Crisp/University of Plymouth: 15; Brian Evans: 27; Fris Imatge: 41, 43; Jan Gehl: 11; Crispin Gill/Western Morning News: 1; Rem Koolhaas/OMA: 21; Patricia & Angus Macdonald: 4, 5, 6; Henri Matisse, *Dance*, 1910 © Succession H. Matisse/DACS 2004: p. 97; MBM Arquitectes: cover, 10, 12, 23, 24, 28, 30, 31, 32, 33, 34, 35, 36, 37, 38, 40, 42, 44, 45, 46, 47, 49, 50, 51, 52, 53, 55, 56, 57, 58, 59, 60, 61, 62, 63, 64, 65, 67, 68, 69, 71, 72, 73, 75; Plymouth City Council: 22, 26, 29, 70, 74; Aldo Rossi: 39; Lloyd Russell/University of Plymouth: 66; SWERDA: 20; University of Plymouth: 2; Wagner & Debes Geographical Institute Leibzig: 7; Watson, J. & Abercrombie, P/Underhill Ltd: 14, 16, 17, 18, 19